PRAISE FOR KARIE CASSELL AND *THE DOMINO DIET*

"A life-changing book that unlocks the secret with a formula to create a wealth of health and success. Karie Cassell brings a twist of humor through stories that you will relate to and will create for you long-lasting results."

— Mary Morrissey, Founder of Brave Thinking Institute

"Karie Cassell has brought her life experience as a dietitian and life coach into the genius of the Domino Diet formula. *The Domino Diet* will be the last book you read to break down paradigms stemming from your food relationships. As a person who has a love-hate relationship with food and was diagnosed with breast cancer, I've had many aha moments reading this book. *The Domino Diet* will help you heal from the inside out by helping you repattern your thoughts to lead to better results. The book is a true answer to so many prayers from people not wanting to follow a diet again and still maintaining great health."

— Edna A Castillo, Founder and CEO of Living Reality Dreams

"Having known and worked with Karie for many years, I have always found her to be very passionate about the role of nutrition in health and chronic disease. She engages, encourages, and empowers her clientele in a holistic approach. This approach has only found greater depth and breadth through her experience and passion for teaching. Her book reflects that experience and passion."

— Dr. Rob Burris, Specialist in Internal Medicine, MD

"After reading *The Domino Diet*, I have a completely different perspective on my body and my health! This book kept me engaged with every chapter, and I truly feel my life as a whole is better for having this new knowledge. *The Domino Diet* isn't just a book—it is a way of life!"

— Tara Killen, LMC, Owner-Truth Mastery Endeavors, Boulder, Colorado

"As a book written out of the desire to have a positive impact on literally everyone, *The Domino Diet* dignifies itself as an absolute game-changer. Its holistic approach and Karie's dedication to actionable methods make this book a must-read. I cannot wait to see the reach it will have."

— Karl Vetter, Psychological Advisor and Change Manager

"As a type one diabetic for thirty-four years, I was referred to Karie through my city's leading diabetic specialist. From the moment Karie and I sat down, it was clear she would refreshingly exceed my expectations. Over the following months, I could hardly believe I was actually texting regular screenshots of my blood sugars to a skilled, caring professional who was giving me pragmatic advice in real-time. I learned principles from Karie I will use every day; more importantly, the tighter blood sugar control will, hopefully, give me more of those days."

— Kenton Dueck, CI Specialist, Canada

"Karie is conscientious and diligent when she assists you. Her energetic use of language makes a difference in how she practices the art of writing and speaking. Karie is passionate. She inspires by helping gently improve your health in ways unique to your experience. Karie enlightens her audiences with personal stories and charismatic charm. This is a woman who is undaunted in venturing beyond the familiar."

— Arlene McDonnell, DMT, VP Toastmaster, Grande Prairie, Alberta

"This book is a destined best-seller and a true paradigm-shifter!"

— Karina Klepach, Founder of Infinite Life Mastery, USA

"I signed up for life coaching with Karie hoping to meet some goals and get my life figured out after feeling like I was in a rut for years. Karie not only helped me *see* what I wanted in life, but she truly coached me to manifest those dreams. My life has changed drastically since working with Karie. Her knowledge and motivation helped me to stay on track with my goals and see life through a different, clearer lens. Since being coached by Karie, I have seen everything in my life start to fall into place, and I was able to purchase my dream property! If you are serious about taking control of your own life and creating the life you have always dreamed of, Karie is your coach!"

— Shannon Hinks, Grande Prairie, Alberta

"Karie Cassell is an extraordinary author, nutritionist, and coach. Her compassionate and enthusiastic approach to health and wellness will help me overcome limitations. This book delivers an abundance of knowledge that anyone would benefit from."

— Donna Howald, ABMNM Practitioner,
Life Mastery Consultant, California

"Karie Cassell has the mind of an experienced dietitian and the heart of a transformational life coach. Her book offers an approach to health and wellness that dives deep to help transform the issues underlying our ineffective dieting patterns and problems. The blend of both dietitian and life coach expertise makes *The Domino Diet* a real game-changer in the genre of diet books. I highly recommend this book to anyone wanting to jump off the dieting treadmill and take control of their weight for good."

— Fawn Winterwood, PhD in Education Policy & Leadership, Ohio

"When I first talked to Karie as a new triathlete, she was eager to tackle the issues at hand and offered confidence with her prognosis. Her supportive way of life coaching helped me complete my first 140.6, full-distance race with confidence. I went from a novice athlete to qualifying for Team USA and World Championships!"

— David Dixon, Triathlete Team USA, Florida

"Karie Cassell is a brilliant Transformational Life Coach! She is wonderfully intuitive, and her concept of The Domino Diet is something the profession of Dietetic can truly benefit from, on top of the amazing impact I foresee amongst clients who truly want to have a healthier life. I admire Karie's experience as a Registered Dietitian and a Transformational Life Coach. She has beautifully combined both in this incredible book, *The Domino Diet*. For people looking for the real solution for their health challenges (any challenges in life, it is the same mindset approach), Karie's teachings will deliver results!"

— Lin Yuan-Su, Success Coach, Registered Dietitian, Speaker

"Chock-full of knowledge and wisdom, *The Domino Diet* casts a fresh new light into nutrition, diet, and health. It's a practical and powerful educational tool to help you live a healthier life through a deeper understanding of the mind-body connection."

— Susan Friedmann, CSP, International Bestselling Author of
Riches in Niches: How to Make it BIG in a small Market

"From macronutrients and munchies to mindfulness and manifesting change, *The Domino Diet* reveals that food and outside forces aren't what's in charge of your health. Each chapter presents strategies, action steps, and engaging stories to help you recognize that healing is an inside job. It does this in part by presenting the word 'diet' in its original meaning: a way of living. Simply put, this is a powerful guidebook to inner pathways to greater health, so that each one of us is better equipped to make lives—including our own—much better."

— Ken Streater, International Best-Selling Author of
Be the Good and *The Gift of Courage*

"If you feel like potato chips are all you have in life to look forward to, you've found the right book. Karie Cassell will get you motivated to turn your life around. This book isn't just about counting calories but understanding what triggers your food cravings and how you can satisfy yourself in ways that don't involve food. *The Domino Diet Formula* will have you knocking down all the dominos that have been sabotaging your success."

— Tyler R. Tichelaar, PhD and award-winning author
of *Narrow Lives* and *The Best Place*

"It's time to end emotional eating and thinking and embrace your destiny to take back control of your life and weight. Karie Cassell will show you how with inspiring stories, practical tools and exercises, and a lot of common sense advice that will have you rethinking your food choices and portions and choosing health and happiness over more Heath bars and hamburgers."

— Patrick Snow, Publishing Coach and International Best-Selling Author of *Creating Your Own Destiny* and *Boy Entrepreneur*

"Karie Cassell has been a registered dietitian for more than thirty years. She has studied nutrition, dieting, and perhaps most importantly, the emotions that affect many of our food choices. In *The Domino Diet Formula*, she shares her hard-earned wisdom with gentleness and understanding. Her words will motivate you to make the changes you have always wanted in ways that may surprise and delight you. Take a chance on this book—you owe it to yourself."

— Nicole Gabriel, Author of *Finding Your Inner Truth* and *Stepping Into Your Becoming*

"A life-changing book that unlocks the secret with a formula to create a wealth of health and success."
— Mary Morrissey, Founder of Brave Thinking Institute

THE DOMINO DIET

HOW TO HEAL YOU FROM THE INSIDE OUT

KARIE CASSELL

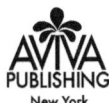

AVIVA PUBLISHING
New York

The Domino Diet: How to Heal You from the Inside Out

Copyright 2021 by Karie Cassell. All rights reserved.

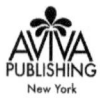

Published by:
Aviva Publishing
Lake Placid, NY
(518) 523-1320

All Rights Reserved. No part of this book may be used or reproduced in any manner whatsoever without the expressed written permission of the author. Address all inquiries to:

Karie Cassell
780-814-2983
info@thedominodiet.com
www.TheDominoDiet.com
www.KLCLifeWise.com

ISBN: 978-1-6361808-6-1(hard cover)
ISBN: 978-1-5136876-6-7 (eBook)
Library of Congress Control Number: 2021906088

Editors: Tyler Tichelaar and Larry Alexander, Superior Book Productions
Cover Designer: Nicole Gabriel, Angel Dog Productions
Author Photo: Tanya Sedore, T. Sedore Photography

Every attempt has been made to properly source all quotes.
Printed in Canada

"Since life is infinite, the concept of an ultimate destiny is inconceivable. When we understand that conciseness is the only reality, we know that it is the only creator. This means that your consciousness is the creator of your destiny."

— Neville (Neville Lancelot Goddard)

"Nothing is impossible. The word itself says 'I'm Possible.'"

— Audrey Hepburn

DEDICATION

To my daughter Seanna. As I always say to you, *What did a mom like me ever do to deserve such a beautiful soul like you?* You are the very reason for me to rise after many falls and the inspiration to write this book and create a legacy. I love you with everything in me. You are the reason I carried on in difficult times and stood firm after falling. You are so gifted and bring a *true* light to everyone. I can only hope I have passed down the wisdom I have discovered to help you continue the healing on this planet. I ask every day what a mom like me ever did to deserve a daughter as beautiful inside and out as you!

To my husband, Stephen Cassell. Thank you for your support and belief in me—for listening to my heart's desires over and over and being a soft place to fall in moments of difficulty. You have taught me about unconditional love. I live deep within life now, no longer on the surface. Your love is a gift. I love you deeply!

To my mom, Julienne Lorenz (also known as Claire): I am so very thankful for the sacrifices you made. You've been my "rudder on a river," balancing me on choppy waters. I am inspired by your growth in worldly wisdom despite your own choppy waters. I also aspire to your class, your beauty, and your centeredness. I love you from the bottom of my heart!

To my dad, Allan Lorenz (also known as Leroy): You have always been a pillar of support and guidance for me. Your unconditional love, your sacrifices, and your wisdom are the backbone of my willingness to strive for more. I would not be a goal-setter with perseverance if it were not for you. I am beyond proud of your *rags to riches* story.

To my best friend, Vonda McDermott: Thank you for your lifelong friendship and forty years of being a partner in believing, for the millions of heart-felt conversations through the journey of our lives, for the tears, cheers, and laughter. You are my sister by heart!

To my brother, Wade Lorenz: Thank you for being the "outside the box" thinker that made it feel normal for me to be me. You are a borderline genius in my book. Thank you for bringing hope to our lives in tumultuous times.

To my bonus boys, Tyler and Riley Cassell: Thank you for teaching me layers of love I would not have been exposed to. You have blessed me in so many ways, teaching so many things I would not have learned without you. I am gifted with two sons thanks to your mom and dad.

To my grandmothers: You have inspired many of the stories in my book. You were both influences. You each modeled the power of women, wisdom, and strength. Grandma, you were always there for me, no matter what. Mémère, I attribute my gift of intuition to you and your current guidance from heaven.

To my sister, Alison Lorenz: I love you more than you will ever know. Thank you for bringing me a perspective of spirituality. Thank you also for the gift of your boys, Jordan and Nathan, who I was able to help raise in earlier years.

Tim Quinn: Thank you for your support over the years, the experiences, and for being such a wonderful father to our daughter! I will always hold you in my heart.

ACKNOWLEDGMENTS

I could not have written this book without inspiration from many sources. Therefore, I wish to express my heartfelt gratitude to the following:

A Course in Miracles, Larry Alexander, Brave Thinking Institute, Danny Bird, John Boggs, Mat Boggs, Rich Boggs, Jules Bourgeois, Lillian Bourgeois, Dr. Rob Burris, Deana Bursey, Paulette Campiou, Stephen Cassell, Juliet Clark, Scott Clement, Rebecca Dietzen, Tony Dietzen, Susan Friedmann, D. Dirsten, Nicole Gabriel, Stan Haugland, Jennifer Jiménez, Lynn Kitchen, Joanne Kriaski, Allan Lorenz, Julienne Lorenz, Erin Lynch, Vonda McDermott, Rob Mclean, Valerie Mills, Mary Morrissey, Al and Justine Newton, Seanna Quinn, Tim Quinn, Dr. Barry Ramaswamy, Christine Richmond, Jared Rosen, Joanne Schweitzer, Ben Shanks, Patrick Snow, Tyler Tichelaar, Dr. Ellen Toth, Marguerite Weaver, Kirsten Welles, Dr. Yolanda Westra, and Lin Yuan-Su.

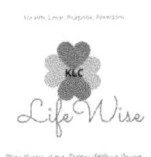

"When health is absent, wisdom cannot reveal itself, strength cannot fight, intelligence cannot be applied, art cannot become manifest, wealth becomes useless."

— Herophilus, Ancient Greek Physician

CONTENTS

Preface: It Wasn't Your Fault — 25

Introduction: Starting Right With New Wisdom — 29

Section 1: The First Domino—Thoughts Makes It Sow — 35

   Chapter 1: Rethinking Diets — 37

      Ritual Revision
      Lighting Your Way
      Fasting Your Diet Thinking
      Filling Your Healing Thinking
      Mind, Spirit, Body: Forgoing Silos

   Chapter 2: Confessions of a Dietitian — 53

      Too Many Plates to Bear
      Keep Spinning or Fail and Fall
      Common Fails in Falls
      "Good" Grief
      Rising in Spring
      The Separation
      Bridging the Gap
      The Domino Diet Formula

   Chapter 3: Understanding Your Two Minds — 71

      Minding Your Mind
      Think and Grow Your Mind
      Your Two Minds
      Empower vs. Willpower

How to "Handle" Your Thoughts
Feeding Your Thoughts
The Science of Growing Your Mind
Food for Thought Cravings

Section 2: The Second Domino—Every Little Breath You Take — 91

Chapter 4: Two Broken Hearts Too Young — 93

Letting Go in Transition
Healing Breathing
"Weighting" to Exhale
You Take My Breath Away

Section 3: The Third Domino—Hormonally Speaking — 105

Chapter 5: Switch Into Thrive — 107

Disordered Eating
Taking Flight
Helpful Hormones
DNA Decoding
No News Is Good Chews
Repatterning
Your Inner Child, Your Inner Beauty
R&R Supplements

Chapter 6: Men-O-Pause — 125

Menopause
Hot Flash!
Manopause
A Midlife Awakening Is Not a Crisis

Section 4: The Fourth Domino—Rising Above   **137**

  Chapter 7: Digesting Your Feelings With Your Friend Jack   **141**
          Daniels

    Trapped and Triggered
    Afraid of Letting Go
    Picking Up Your Good Vibrations
    Transforming Your Attitude Altitude
    From Worrier to Warrior
    Should or Should Not

  Chapter 8: Exposing Your Fears   **157**

    Four Barriers to Success

  Chapter 9: Love Hertz   **165**

    Love Layers
    Addicted to Love
    Discovering Your True Cravings
    That's Your Story—Are You Sticking to It?

Section 5: Between the Fourth and Fifth Domino—Trans-   **179**
      forming You

  Chapter 10: Finding Your Freedom   **183**

    Driving Out of Balance
    Assessing Your Balance
    Defining Burnout
    Making a "You" Turn
    Need a Tow?

Chapter 11: Surviving the School of Hard Knocks   197

Boxing With Destiny
Paradigms 101
Schooling on Change
Turning Adversity Into Your University
A Course in Transformation

Chapter 12: What Do Veggies and Forgiveness Have in Common?   211

Bittersweet: Being Bitter or Better
Double-Dipping
Speaking for Love or Eating for Fear

Section 6: The Fifth Domino—Stepping Into Your Authentic You   223

Chapter 13: Uncovering Cravings   227

Breakfast to Break-the-Fast
Craving Checklist
Uni-Tasking

Chapter 14: Banishing Body Shame and the Hunger Game   239

Balancing the Scales
Trading Yo-Yos for Dominos
Portion Distortion
Learning to Hand Jive
Hunger Helper
The Eater's Digest: Morning Starts at Night

Chapter 15: Your Foundation   **261**

    Wholly Macros
    Drinking Water Works
    Java Junction
    It's Not Pasta's Fault

Chapter 16: Arming Up With Micronutrients   **273**

    Flexitarian
    Putting the Heal Back Into Health
    Healing From the Inside Out
    Micronutrient-Packed Meals
    Micronutrient Robbers

Chapter 17: Understanding the Five Ws of Supplements   **287**

    The Armor of Iron
    The Protein Combo
    Grandma's Pharmacy
    Nature's Pantry
    Immune-Boosting Agents
    The Rise and Fall of Apples

Chapter 18: Staying Resilient   **303**

    Ordinary to Extraordinary: Top Ten Tips
    Mindshift
    Healing With Heels
    Your True Benefits
    Weathering "Storms" With Support

Chapter 19: Calendarizing — 317

    Assess, Adapt, Correct
    Poor Mondays
    Wishing or Kissing
    Happy New Year
    It's a Brand-New Day
    App for That
    Turning a Year Around

Section 7: The Sixth Domino—Embracing Your Results — 333

Chapter 20: Lost and Found Weight — 337

    Maintenance Mindset: A "Wealth of Health"
    Prescription to Maintaining Health
    Common Chronic Diseases
    Practicing and Mastering
    Mastermind Mentor
    Your Invisible Voice
    Out of the Blue
    Be, Do, Have vs. Have, Be, Do
    Learning a New Language to Mind-Full Results
    Connecting the Dots
    The Healer in You

A Final Note: Your Optimal Well-Being — 363
About the Author — 369
About KLC Lifewise Coaching — 373
Book Karie Cassell to Speak at Your Next Event — 375

"The lamps are different but the light is the same."

— Rumi

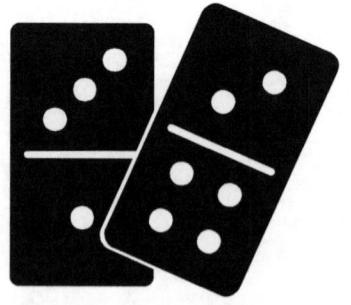

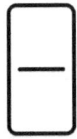

PREFACE: IT WASN'T YOUR FAULT

"Only the healed mind can experience revelation with lasting effect."

— *A Course in Miracles*

It was all backward! For decades, your symptoms have been treated at the symptom level, leaving the root cause missed and your symptoms continuing and unresolved. You have probably tried and failed, and tried and failed again, leaving you feeling hopelessly flawed, lost, and burned out. Do you feel like a sinking ship? Have you bailed water to the point of exhaustion? Do you keep bailing or look for the cause instead?

If you are unhappy with your health or weight, something started the ball in motion long before your emotional eating and food relationship battles. If you have a diagnosis, again, things occurred long before your disease turned into a disease. Truthfully, your emotions are somewhere in the middle of the sequence of events. The focus, up until now, has been at the end, on diets and pills as the main solution. Has that been working? Have pills and diets provided you with more freedom or misfortune? Who prospers from your misfortune? Who wins despite all your efforts while you are left feeling emptier? In these pages, not only will you discover that the source of your leaks is the diet cycles you have endured, but you will also find a guide to your freedom!

Imagine a dominos game with the pieces all in a row. Each one is aligned precisely. All it will take is one flick of a finger for a chain reaction to occur—the right momentum and perfect timing will knock every domino down to the very end, creating a "domino effect." But what happens if the dominos are spaced too far apart or one is missing? What happens if you start at the end after all the pieces fall and you try pushing them the opposite way? Is it better to start at the beginning or the end?

Your thoughts are like those dominos, the beginning of your world internally and externally! Internally, they activate a rhythm to your breathing and switch on specific hormonal responses. Depending on the hormones prompted by your breathing, your body chemistry responds accordingly, in a cadence that can influence your actions. Your actions produce your results, good or bad, internally and externally. Like a series of fallen dominos, a whole series of events took place long before you began to experience your current results or symptoms.

The Domino Diet is a simple, innovative guide. It offers a formula to return you to health. While some circumstances may seem out of your control, leaving you circling round and round, when you connect to your thought world, you will discover the root cause of your symptoms or illness. Awareness of your thoughts will help you begin managing your symptoms, disease, weight battles, and more. By focusing on your thoughts, you will discover you have more control than you "think." In these pages, as I reveal what you can do, you will move from hopeless to hopeful. Truthfully, there is so much more you can do to finally create results you will love. Starting with your thoughts, we will explore all aspects of this formula, which looks like this:

The Domino Diet Formula

Thoughts⇒ Breath⇒ Hormones⇒ Feelings⇒ Action⇒ Results⇒ Freedom

The stories in this book are based on real individuals, whose names have been changed to protect them. Like you, they tried time and time again to achieve their desired results, only to end up more disheartened than they were from the start. Discovering The Domino Diet Formula not only helped them achieve optimal wellness, but they discovered the gift of discovering their authentic self and produced "wealth" in all areas of their lives, including their health!

Each chapter will provide you with the opportunity to reflect and customize your journey. Action steps are provided to allow you to absorb and apply your discoveries at your own pace. To optimize your experience, I recommend reading one chapter a day. That way you can reflect upon and "digest" the information in it.

Are you ready to start feeling better? Are you ready to meet and exceed your health goals, stop sabotaging yourself, and enjoy balance and a feeling of fulfillment? I hope you are. I hope you will take this journey with me now.

Let's begin.

Karie Cassell

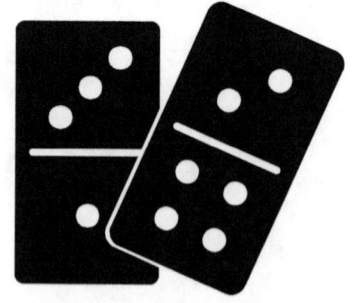

INTRODUCTION:
STARTING RIGHT WITH NEW WISDOM

> "The time will come when the work of the physician will not be to treat and attempt to heal the body, but to heal the mind, which in turn will heal the body. The true physician will be a teacher; his work will be to keep the people well, instead of attempting to make them well after sickness and disease has come on."
>
> — Ralph Waldo Trine

You have tried everything. One minute you are told to eat this way and the next you are told it was all wrong. You might say, "Why try? Nothing seems to work anyway. And as soon as I lose it, I seem to sabotage it anyway." Meanwhile, diet propaganda continues to drive a billion-dollar market with a mere 3 percent success rate, while disease and weight issues are more prevalent than ever before.

Who benefits? Who decides what you should look like or weigh? It seems to be a moving target. Even the "perfect" images we are trained to aspire to are usually airbrushed pictures of hungry, unhappy people. The flawed diet industry makes you feel flawed, guilty, and shunned for being hungry. Yet we have a primal instinct and need to eat, but with more rules than ever before. It's time to end this way. The fight is over! You deserve more than food "battles" and mixed messages. No more "delusions with illusions." At a 3 percent success, their way is clearly not working.

But what does work, especially with your busy schedule on top of it all? Between balancing home, work, time, and money, you are exhausted, and then you have to be chef and maid too? The time finally arrives for your workday to end. You get ready to put your feet up, but instead, you have to figure out what to eat and what to feed your family. You need to figure out what is healthy and what is not. Plus, after dinner, you'll need to decide if you have time to exercise. The whirlwind can leave you stressed, with the pressure ever dialing upward while your self-esteem dials downward.

I feel your pain. I have been there too. I was constantly trying to be the perfect mother, spouse, sister, daughter, and dietitian with the perfect life, but on the inside, I was suffocating. Then, when my world of "rules" crumbled, there were no more dangling carrots, never mind wanting carrots to replace chips; chips were all I had to look forward to. Life and a proper diet were easy when the white picket fence was up, but when the storm came and blew it all down, I wanted to run and hide, and not with a salad or vegetables and hummus. I wanted comfort food—chips, please, with a side of chocolate and wine. Oh, and make that a double. I was not born a dietitian; I was born a human, after all. In the end, though, eating badly only made matters worse and caused more battles.

You may have recently been diagnosed with a chronic disease. You may have lost weight and regained weight so many times you're scared to get your hopes up to try again. Maybe you succeed at first, only to have self-sabotage win in the end. What if I told you there might be something else going on and your weight issue may not be your fault or the real problem? It is likely something was not only missing but completely backward.

In the chapters ahead, you will learn how your mind operates for and against you. You will see how some of your habits formed before you were even born and how they can affect your choices today. You have reasons for self-sabotage, but once you see the connections, you will be empowered to override them. While you cannot chase away the darkness, you can turn on a light. You will learn how to claim your power, gain the *will-to-empower* rather than just willpower, and end emotional eating and thinking. You will learn who truly commands your choices. You will discover you have a switch in your mind's control center that will allow the pieces to fall into place the right way and connect to all areas of your life. You will begin to conquer emotional battles with food, understand cravings, and your hidden barriers to success.

You are equipped with more than you know. Of course, you may not believe me; you may have lost hope, not knowing whom to trust. I get that. But I promise you this—if you lean in, you will be shown a new way to come out of *disease* and into the ease of health-harmony. You can trust the tools are within you and will emerge more and more as you release old patterns while installing new ones. You will renew and discover what you are really *hungry* for, and you will discover the *true* you.

If you apply the wisdom, strategies, techniques, and research offered in this book, you will achieve the promise of the subtitle: *How to Heal You from the Inside Out!*

As a registered dietitian for more than thirty years who has studied both traditional and non-traditional medicine, I can help you navigate through the pitfalls of media hype and provide you with true health messages. I have worked with thousands of clients to uncover what works and does not work, how to set goals, how to measure genuine successes, and how to veer away from self-sabotage. Plus, I will help you discover where your fear of success comes from—it goes back further than you might think. After decades of witnessing fad diets, trends, and the war on macronutrients, I will help familiarize you with your hidden army of skills and micronutrients to help revitalize and conquer your food battles. As a certified life coach, I will help you connect all areas of your life while busting paradigms and old patterns that no longer serve you.

While I do not have all the answers, I promise to provide you with realistic, repeatable, and reliable ways to start again the right way. What used to be a simple time to gather at meals has become consumed with guilt and complexity, as though you must be a detective for your plate. How could you have known how to start right with all the jargon to trudge through? What if it can be simple again? What if the pressure valve was released, allowing you to enjoy food as it was intended? Your ancestors paved the way for you to have the abundance of today, and now you are made to feel guilty for enjoying it? You deserve a better alternative. I am a dietitian on a mission to bring back the true meaning of the word diet—to *put the "heal" back into health* and remove the "stinking thinking" that took it out in the first place. I have come to realize there is no ceiling on the possibilities of self-development. And I know for sure there is no such thing as perfection. But progress is always possible, and I will help you progress.

Hope is in your hands in the form of this guide to renewal, even if you have been lost a dozen or more times before. I know you will discover something new. I believe this with all my heart—the system cannot fail once you awaken to it and apply it.

I want to celebrate you! You are in the right place. You have stepped toward opportunity and results that you will love. You have made a "U-turn" toward your *true* health and a new beginning with a positive end in mind. You will dial up your desires, by putting the pieces in the right order with easy steps to freedom. You can have a "wealth of health" using a holistic approach and never have to "diet" again.

Would you like to find the missing pieces? As a dietitian, life coach, and someone who has been there, I will mentor and support you on your journey with *The Domino Diet*. Are you ready to step outside the box? Are you ready to align and expand your comfort zone and become an achiever of goals and dreams? Let's get started and make this journey together. Dear diamond, it is your time to shine. Let's go!

The Domino Diet Formula

Thoughts⇒ Breath⇒ Hormones⇒ Feelings⇒ Actions⇒ Results⇒ Freedom

> It's not about the diet and it doesn't start or end with the diet either. What are you really hungry for?

> "What the caterpillar calls the end of the world, the master calls a butterfly."
>
> — Richard Bach

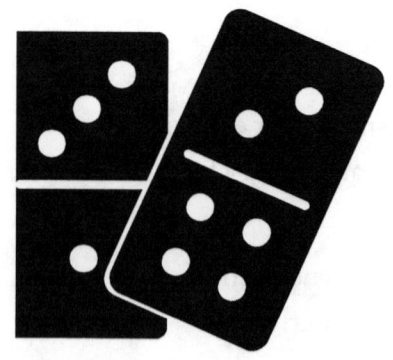

SECTION 1

THE FIRST DOMINO— THOUGHTS MAKES IT SOW

The Domino Diet Formula: Thoughts

Thoughts⇒ Breath⇒ Hormones⇒ Feelings⇒ Actions⇒ Results⇒ Freedom

"Thoughts are like seeds; they all have energy. The subconscious knows no difference, and it goes to work to grow what you sow."

— Mary Morrissey

You live in a thought world where ideas and thoughts are a form of currency. The moment you have a thought, it is yours "in the making" according to how you invest your thinking. How you invest your thinking determines your returns. Scholars and authors have long said if you think positive thoughts, you receive positive results. If you think negative thoughts, you receive negative results. Either way, you reap what you sow.

Do you tend more often to think positively or negatively? What about the thoughts in the background you are not always aware of? How do they sow?

We'll explore these questions in this section.

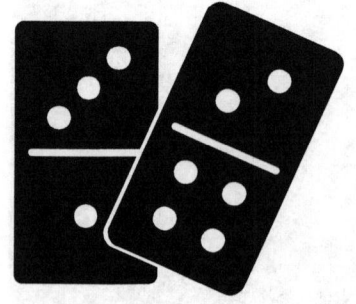

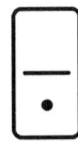

CHAPTER 1
RETHINKING DIETS

"Falling down is not failure. Failure comes when you stay where you have fallen."

— Socrates

Pamela stood at her kitchen sink for what felt like hours. Her mind moved a "mile a minute," trying to assess whether she should move to the phone and call *911* or stay for fear of falling on the way. She could feel dizziness overtake her as the lights in her home formed a vortex of swirling stars, as if to pull her seductively down a dark tunnel. The noise from the TV muffled the sound of her heart pounding louder and faster. The fear of something happening to her alone in her home only enhanced the symptoms. What started as a nosebleed became a full-on panic attack. *What is going on here? Am I going to die alone? Is this a heart attack?* she thought. As time passed, dehydration triggered hot flashes, drenching her hair and clothes, creating more dehydration and more hot flashes! Pamela had no idea if her hormones or a panic attack or both were responsible.

Pamela had experienced hot flashes before, but a panic attack was completely new to her. She was on medication for high blood pressure, and her doctor had advised her to lose weight. Still, her weekend was filled with forbidden pleasures since extreme loneliness seemed even worse. This time, though, her body spoke louder to get her attention. Something had to change for her to find freedom outside the cage holding her back from what she truly craved.

Like many, Pamela spent her weekend sitting on the couch with little movement, watching TV while eating junk foods. Nothing was unusual about this routine. She lived alone, and it gave her something to look forward to. This time, though, her gushing nosebleed had sent her running to the nearest sink. With bent arms and gripped hands, she drooped her head over the sink while attempting to poise and elevate pressures in her now aching back along with shifting her swollen cramped legs. Her awkwardly perched position did give her a bird's-eye view of the crime scene and its evidence—empty chip bags, mini-chocolate bars, and take-out containers.

Eventually, Pamela made it back to her couch, where she sat dizzily assessing her situation. Out of sheer desperation, after the fall from her perch, this broken bird needed something to grab ahold of.

Imagine you are falling off a cliff. Are you hopelessly reaching for anything to break your fall? In desperation, you grab the smallest branch, despite knowing it may not hold you for long. Unfortunately, diet propaganda knows how to play you during your dire times, presenting you with an olive branch that often ends up a mere twig.

Pamela signed on for yet another diet program—a small branch to hold with promises of quick weight loss if adhering to its ways. Now even more anxious, she locked herself further in her cage with new routines of salads and magic potions to fit society's mold. When friends invited her out, she declined from fear of giving into temptation—a paradox really since longing for companionship was the perpetrator of her decline in the first place. Now, her loneliness was replaced by a diet regimen.

Diet programs have convincing "all or nothing," "my way or the highway" language and imply, "If you fail, it's your fault." They do not advise you on how to deal with feelings and, if you fall, they leave you and your feelings to pick up the pieces. Plus, they often approach things backward, suggesting you will be happy after losing weight. They claim to know what will make you happy as you attempt to prop things into place, but they still leave you with missing pieces in their one-size-fits-all strategies.

While Pamela did, in the next five months, lose fifty pounds, it was not the first time she had lost weight. Concurrently, though, she unexpectedly lost her mother, with whom she was extremely close. They had shared weekly visits and phone calls, and her mother had provided support through Pamela's divorce. Everything escalated again for Pamela with her mom gone. Her diet could not withstand the stress, which inevitably triggered a reunion for her with what she could depend on: chips and dip.

Pamela's hot flashes intensified, which meant more sleepless nights from soaked bedsheets waking her. Now awake, her mind set off the worry fiasco: How will I pay the bills? Will I always be alone? What am I doing wrong?

Habits are like that. They do not come with neon signs; they creep in like creatures in the night. Not knowing how to cope, Pamela's weight crept back and carried with it more shame. Now her mission to lose weight in hopes of attracting her lifelong partner was replaced with a lifelong weight battle. Instead of falling off a cliff, she felt kicked off. Even more hopeless than before, she had no idea where to start. How can you fix something when you do not know where the problem begins or ends? Fixing your life problems with a diet alone is like bailing water without looking for the leak. The bailing keeps you so busy that you are distracted from what you are really longing for. While focused on the problem, you can lose sight of solutions. It only works one way. Pamela was not actually hungry for food but for freedom outside her cage.

> "You can't see that I'm hurting. You don't notice the pain. It feels like everyone is sitting in sunshine while I drown in the rain."
>
> — Unknown

RITUAL REVISION

Pamela was a product of her upbringing. While she was growing up, her mother was "always" on a diet. She remembers her mother trying on clothes and saying, "I look ugly," and "I look fat." Her mother did not know any better; her generation didn't talk about loving your body. Most didn't. Pamela's mother grew up on a farm where the morning rituals involved feeding seven kids. The closest they came to "take care of your body" was to form a line for a teaspoon of cod liver oil once a week. This was a time when home baking was still in the making and fast foods were leftovers heated in a pan. Food was functional for physical strength, and scales only existed in the doctor's office. Then, suddenly, the bathroom scale entered every home as the new measuring tool, but it didn't come with an interpreter to translate the numbers. The learning curve, unfortunately, was driven by TV and friends who would lead most people to a state of "compare and despair."

Pamela and her husband each had stressful jobs working long hours. Over time, she sensed challenges in their relationship. To offset this, they started meeting Fridays at their favorite Italian restaurant to connect their "passing ships." They became two "foodies" enjoying pasta, fine wines, and decadent desserts. Saturdays were spent busily with housework, but they developed a movie night with a popcorn routine, and on Sundays, they caught up with family over dinner. Monday, though, the morning ritual began with Pamela weighing herself—at which point the deliciousness of a romantic weekend to salvage a marriage faded into the growing numbers on the scale. A downward spiral of low self-esteem and depression took over despite a weekend most would envy. When she arrived at work, Pamela's coworkers would ask, "How was your weekend?" "Fine," she would say. Despite the hours of loving connection, the two seconds on the scale outweighed it all. Soon, she stopped her relationship routine on behalf of her weighing routine, but as a result, the passing ships continued passing until their marriage ended.

Losing relationships became an underlying theme for Pamela. As a child of divorce, in her opinion, she had lost her father to another family. Previous boyfriends had left her for someone else, and now, her husband had too. With her mother gone, things felt out of Pamela's control, losing her love of food in times of loneliness was unconsciously another loss she did not want to undertake, but it came with a price and she needed to find a new way.

LIGHTING YOUR WAY

"Darkness cannot drive out darkness; only light can do that."

— Martin Luther King, Jr.

Imagine you are standing in a large department store searching for a lamp. After searching the rows and rows of lamps of different shapes and sizes, you find the perfect one and bring it home. Setting it down, you plug it in, and voilà, your dark corner is now lit! You notice, now and then, though, that your lamp flickers, then dims, and then brightens again. As time passes, it dims even more until suddenly your light goes out. Like a private detective, you inspect your lamp, turning it upside down, looking for cracks and flaws. You lift the shade, twist the bulb, and double-check the plug. After scratching your head, you realize there must be something else. Finally, you have *a light bulb moment,* and you make your way to the breaker panel. Sure enough, the breaker flipped. You flip the switch and proudly proceed to your bright room. However, the dim, flickering light show starts all over again. Only this time, you hear "buzz-zap!" and your light goes out. With the help of your electrician friend, you find, "You have a flaw in your power cord."

Do you feel like Pamela? Does your light flicker and dim? Have you tried everything but nothing works? Do you check your lamp, or is there another root cause?

Most diets and medical procedures treat your symptoms but miss your entire circuitry. Diabetes, obesity, digestive disorders, and so on require more than repeatedly replacing a bulb. They require an electrician friend—someone who can look much deeper and find the root cause. You need a holistic approach that encompasses the breaker panel, outlet, cord, lamp, bulb, and all. I am not pointing fingers since, as a dietitian for more than thirty years, I have also said, "What are your symptoms? Here is your diet. What are your symptoms? Here is your pill." That was a pill, diet, pill, diet, flicker that not only burned you out but burnt me out as well—until I discovered new tools.

"The power that makes the body, heals the body."

— Dr. Joe Dispenza

FASTING YOUR DIET THINKING

"You cannot solve a problem with the level of thinking that caused the problem."

— Albert Einstein.

Have you lived with symptoms for so long that they feel normal? Do they seem to pull you into the habit of ailment thinking? Have you heard conversations where everyone seems to be competing to see who has it worst? The trouble is that the solution to a problem does not exist on the same level as the problem, so solving it requires a new way of thinking and being. The solutions to symptoms are on two different frequencies, much like two channels on your TV. If your thinking is driven by *The Diet Channel* broadcasting sacrifice and restrictions, you might want to change channels.

Some dieters are eating 400-1,000 calories a day, making it nearly impossible to meet you're nutritional needs or sustain health, let alone heal symptoms. Unfortunately, impressionable teens are also following these diets, causing growth, hormone, and metabolism errors that can develop into diseases that can follow them into adulthood. Think of a time you followed a restricted diet. Is it possible it contributed to your struggles today? You may have even heard a small voice suggesting your diet was unhealthy, but the dangling carrot of a size two continued to lure you. How did it get this way? Who decides what you should look like and how to get there?

The word "diet" comes from the Greek word origin *diaita*, which means "a way of life." Did you catch that? A way of life. Diets today hardly seem to be a way of life. Many are painstaking, temporary, and line the pockets of companies while robbing yours, especially in desperate times. While some diets can help provide a path to health, diseases like diabetes, obesity, heart disease, cancers, and digestive disorders are still on the rise. Wouldn't there be a downward trend if they worked? Many diets even come with disclaimers like "not recommended for children" or "not recommended during pregnancy," which hardly sounds like a way of life. What will it take to stop this harmful diet thinking?

The *true* meaning of diet needs to make a comeback. This was my intention for the word *diet* in the title of this book. It is time to change channels and stop repeating unhealthy eating and dieting thinking. It isn't working!

> "Insanity: Doing the same thing over and over again and expecting different results."
>
> — Albert Einstein

First, it may help to uncover and dismiss the images we see every day and everywhere that suggest we should look and dress a certain way. These "perfect" snapshots of life require professional makeup artists, airbrushing, and restricted diets. The models appear to be happy, but are they?

Chasing images on TV is like chasing a moving target. Not long ago, Marylin Monroe was the ideal woman. The famous model had voluptuous curves in a size twelve and represented the essence of "sexy." Yet her ending suggests she was unhappy. Today, we'd say she was overweight. Back then, if she had lost twenty pounds of her luxurious curves, the headlines would have declared, "Marilyn Monroe Is Dying!" Can we dispense with letting magazines and Hollywood *teach* us about *happiness*?

Second, restricted diets are counterproductive to true healing. Your body will not effectively build muscle, repair itself, or provide optimal vitality if deficient in nourishment. In fact, extreme calorie restrictions can induce mood swings, lower immune systems, and hormonal fluctuations, otherwise known as imbalances. If you were stranded on a desert island with inadequate food, your metabolism would lower to preserve your vital organs. If you try to lose weight or manage a diagnosis with "old diet thinking," your metabolism might continue running old patterns too.

A revision is ahead for you, though. No more Monday weigh-in rituals with a side-order of guilt and punishment. It is time to lose your diet thinking and start your healing thinking. As Sophia Loren, another famous model and actress, said, "Beauty is how you feel inside, and it reflects in your eyes. It is not something physical."

FILLING YOUR HEALING THINKING

"You have the power to heal yourself, and you need to know. We think so often that we are helpless, but we're not. We always have the power of our minds. Calmly and consciously use your power."

— Louise Hay

Suzy Prudden, a mind-body-fitness expert, suggests healing the body requires the power of the mind and using the four key concepts listed below—taken with some modifications from the *Brave Thinking Institute: Life Mastery Consultant Training Manual.*

1. Nurture your body with the *right thoughts*—love your body and it will love you.
2. Nurture your body with the *right food*—fuel your body with whole, fresh, unprocessed foods.
3. Nurture your body with the *right people*—surround yourself with positive support.
4. Nurture your body with the *right environment*—fresh air, scenery, nature, aromas.

How does someone in optimal health go about their day? Do they think positively? How does a healed body stay healed? If you heal with new habits but return to old, unhealthy habits, will the disease return? A healed mind is more likely to create a healed body. An unhappy mind will likely produce disease. Even if you must *fake it 'til you make it*, begin to match your mind to the result you are looking for; you will become the result you are longing for.

A diet high in antioxidants, healthy fatty acids, and fiber, along with long walks in nature, promotes health and can conquer most diseases. This isn't news though, so why aren't most people following this routine?

Sadly, some believe in their pain and ailments almost to the extent that they are part of their identity. Unfortunately, when we focus on ailments, it is difficult to think positively. We can change this thinking by recognizing the truth in our thinking.

For instance, if you have arthritis in your left hand, are you unhealthy everywhere? If you lose an arm, are you unhealthy? What you focus on grows. Focusing and saying, "I am so unhealthy" will continue to produce unhealthy thinking. It may be hard to believe, but for some, sickness serves them—somehow and quite possibly in-part what holds them back from implementing what they know to be healthier ways, as I mentioned earlier.

Filling yourself with the desire to heal and have optimal well-being starts with the mind telling the body and not the other way around.

> "Healing involves an understanding of what the illusion of sickness is for. Healing is impossible without this. Healing is accomplished the instant the sufferer no longer sees the value in pain."
>
> — *A Course in Miracles*

MIND, SPIRIT, BODY: FORGOING SILOS

At what age did you discover you have a body? Were you like most kids waking up with messy hair and thinking nothing of it? Did your parent have to tell you to clean up and brush your teeth? As a kid, I didn't even realize I had a body with flaws, nor did I think to look for them. I was told, "You look like your mom," and "You have your dad's hands," which all seemed flattering enough. I lived in an imaginary world with Barbie and her motorhome, thinking I might one day look that beautiful too. My mother's beauty made me think it was possible. I didn't see that my physique would never measure up—mainly because I hadn't noticed it yet. I just distracted myself with Barbie in her pink Corvette driving into the imaginary sunset.

I was ten and returning from a vacation when someone said, "Hmm, it looks like you gained a few pounds." I instantly felt naked and ashamed for the first time and wanted to cover up and hide—like Eve after biting into the forbidden fruit. I noticed my body, at least in terms of vanity, for the first time, and I saw it as flawed.

When did you notice your body? Did you live in an imaginary mind-world in your youth? Maybe in your teens you focused on your body? In your twenties and thirties, with college or a first job, you may have paid more attention to your mind. Between thirty and forty, you might have vacillated between concentrating on your body and your mind after putting your body through a rendering process like having kids. If you have already reached your forties or fifties, you might have noticed your body changing, but the same vanity no longer propels you. However, vitality begins to be the primary concern. In the awakening of being over fifty, you might ask, "Is there more to life?" and seek more spiritually.

Throughout life, your mind, body, and spirit seem to be treated as disconnected silos. If you felt shame or flawed in your body as a child, you didn't have a developed mind to help you heal. Even today, if you struggle with physical symptoms, you see your family doctor. With mental disorders, you see a different, specialized practitioner. For guidance in spirituality, you seek yet another isolated source.

Wallace Wattles, author of several books including the well-known, 1910 bestseller *The Science of Getting Rich*, said:

> There are three motives for which we live: we live for the body; we live for the mind; we live for the soul. No one of these is better or holier than the other; all are alike desirable, and no one

of the three…can live fully if either of the others is cut short of full life and expression. It is not right or noble to live only for the soul and deny mind or body, and it is wrong to live for intellect and deny body or soul.

What if the *mind, spirit,* and *body* were treated equally together, with all three present in every aspect of life, including your health? The Universe does not favor oxygen over carbon dioxide; it relies on an equal value exchange system with both. Similarly, the exchange system within your mind creates your outer world, and your outer world nourishes your inner world. Your inner world relies on your outer world to feed it, and your outer world requires your inner world to create the desire to seek new experiences.

Your mind, spirit, and body are all connected in an exchange system operating in harmony unless one of those three *slip* into a silo. Your body is like the lamp, your mind like the wiring, and the electricity is your spirit. All three are required for each to operate, and they are intended to work in harmony. Many remedies only focus on the body and neglects the rest of the circuitry. A holistic approach is needed for healing because all of you needs to be healed.

Is this true healing?

Let's connect the mind, spirit, and body as one circuit for true, whole healing and forgo the silos.

REFLECTIONS

1. Have you followed a restricted diet? What was your experience? Why do you no longer follow it?

2. Describe times when your mind, body, and spirit seemed separate or misaligned.

ACTION STEP

Write down your health history. Note any patterns that connected to times of happiness or stress, times like your wedding or planning and going on a trip. Did happiness create better health? What about stress? Experiment with ways you can connect your mind, spirit, and body as one toward health harmony. Go for a walk. Do yoga or dance. When you consciously breathe deeply while walking, does it help clear your mind? Does it cause you to de-stress? Keep notes on your experiences.

SUMMARY

While the word "diet" originally meant "a way of life," the meaning certainly changed over time. Its current meaning has created a billion-dollar industry that fuels our confusion. Many diet claims are built on sacrifices and cycles leading to little improvement in chronic disease trends. Even the better diets are focused on bodily symptoms, but you are more than a body alone. You are mind, spirit, and body, and when you connect your elements inclusively, you can help put the *heal* back into *health*.

In the following pages, you will discover how Pamela and others switched their thinking around, starting with healthy thinking, and discovered what their true needs were. It is time to rewire and free yourself from diet thinking and recharge your healing thinking too. Until you are working with all of your internal elements—mind, body, and spirit—holistically, you are only healing a part of you. This is not true healing. You deserve more! Your failure and fall with diets were not your fault. A true diet is a way of life. It is time to find better educators for something as significant in everyday life as our diets. It is time to put healing thinking first. No more Monday morning rituals defining you.

Are you ready to install a new way of thinking? A new formula?

AFFIRMATION

I am mind, spirit, and body connected harmoniously with my inner and outer world.

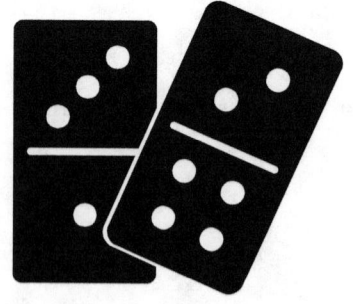

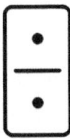

CHAPTER 2
CONFESSIONS OF A DIETITIAN

"You must change your mind, not your behaviour, and this is a matter of willingness. You do not need guidance except at the mind level where change is possible. Change does not mean anything at the symptom level, where it cannot work. Willingness is the only way to make real progress."

— *A Course in Miracles, Transformation*

Wellness has been my calling, my vocation for more than forty years. At thirteen, I thought it was normal to read the *Nutrition Almanac* like it was *Vogue* magazine. I didn't read novels, but the almanac grabbed my attention. My parents were distributors for a supplement company, and therefore, I was surrounded by shelves of vitamins. I loved learning the role of nutrients like vitamin E, lecithin, beta-carotene, etc. I was hooked, and *alternative medicine* became my first real job.

Like a sponge for anything nutrition-related, I cultivated a deep curiosity that led me to a thirty-year career as a *registered dietitian*. It was my purpose and passion all rolled into one. For me, the word *heal* inside the word health stood out like bold print. Hearing the word health was like slipping on a pair of fuzzy, warm slippers I could walk in all day. I wanted nothing more than to be a role model for health, and to do so, I went so far as to run marathons.

Being in peak health and teaching health was a perfect duet, until it wasn't! Everything was great until the floor fell out from under me, taking my health with it. I went from a walking message for dietitians to the poster child for a dietitian's mess.

I stood in the shower with the water beating down, unable to bring myself to step out. With the water still running, I completely collapsed into an awkward, uncomfortable, fetal position with my head cradled into my arms. The shower at least dampened the sound of my uncontrollable blubbering as I purged a flood of tears from my convulsing body—a pile of limbs, skin, and fat with crevasses filled with unrecognized parts. I felt shame and wore a badge that read "Guilty." "What was I thinking?" played over and over like a broken record in my mind.

I did my best to place blame elsewhere, but as I lay there, I realized I was responsible for my mess. In less than six months, I had gone from peak fitness to gaining thirty pounds. My self-esteem spiraled along with everything I had built. The marathoner ran away, and my good days went with her. I wanted a fast way out and had suicidal thoughts, but that would hurt my daughter, who was already reeling from her father and I separating. My love for her stopped me.

TOO MANY PLATES TO BEAR

The "Majestic Plate Spinner" was a captivating act. She was like an octopus, spinning and balancing several plates simultaneously. Each hand propped skinny poles with stacks of spinning plates on top. Between her toes were more poles with more plates. Even on top her head, more plates spun effortlessly. Everyone watched with anticipation, wondering how long she could continue. Then along came the "Dancing Bear," who clumsily danced around her. You could tell they were a new "duo" since when he came along, he seemed to distract her. The bear began weaving between the circles on the floor separating them. Then, with an awkward pirouette, he landed in her circle, managing to graze her elbow, which sent plates flying and crashing one by one…all her hard work, juggling career and home…*smash! smash! smash!* Broken pieces scattered across the floor. After years of training, all it took was one brush with the Bear. Humiliated, embarrassed, and broken, she fled the stage into an iron cocoon.

Are you trying to keep it all together? Have you been through one of the big Ds: Divorce, Diagnosis, or Death of a loved one?

It appears no one is exempted from a brush with misfortune. Loss of a job, betrayal, a loved one who won't speak to you—they are all losses and have within them rightful grief. Divorce is a form of death. Despite how common divorce has become, this form of death comes with negative feelings and finger-pointing from both sides. Many divorces come with yelling and certainly without a praising eulogy. No matter who left whom, both will experience grief.

With a loss of any kind, there is a temptation to fast-track through the process, thereby losing the lessons the loss is supposed to teach. Bypassing grief can leave you split in two with one part holding you back with guilt for not trying harder and the other using anger to pull you forward—leaving claw marks along the way. It's kind of like driving with one foot on the gas and the other on the brake while using the rearview mirror for directions. You end up stuck.

KEEP SPINNING OR FAIL AND FALL

Before her divorce, the Majestic Plate Spinner traveled every weekend with her act. She and her husband agreed to her six-year contract. She would be busy temporarily but with long-term gains that would catapult her career and offer financial freedom in the end. The benefits appeared to outweigh the costs. Everything looked manageable from their vantage point, but unfortunately, the view before the climb was very different than the view from the top. It was like watching your friends standing on the high diving board from below compared to standing up there yourself.

She and her spouse grew apart during her travels to performances. Others went through divorces, but when it was her turn, it all came crashing down. Following right behind her, was the dancing bear, and the once separate acts became a duo. Unlike the *Cirque du Soleil* they thought it would be, they looked more like two clumsy sumo wrestlers thrashing. What happens when two people are failing and falling? Do they hold each other up or push each other down? These two did both.

It was not intentional or part of the plan. She had married her high school sweetheart. They did what everyone did: get married, have kids, and be happy. When she asked for a divorce, it seemed the whole town became judge and jury with court being held in her backyard. The ruling was "guilty," of course, and her prison served platters of humble pie.

The dancing bear and plate spinner married. Still, in stressful times, she tried her usual career runaway tactics like working long hours. In other words, she had not properly grieved first before taking on more with a new relationship. However, fear of another failed marriage convinced her to wear an apron uniform instead, but it was suffocating and left her lifeless and sitting catatonic for hours. Eventually, her self-loathing created internal stress and pushed her into menopause at forty—she was one hot mess.

Why is it some individuals breeze through circumstances, while others get hauled through a wringer? Is there something else going on? Maybe there are a few lessons to be learned from the failures and falls of the Majestic Plate Spinner.

COMMON FAILS IN FALLS

1. Staying busy to distract from what is really failing and falling.
2. Being distracted by looking at someone else's backyard instead of your own.
3. Handing your power over to others so they can push you into a fall.
4. Getting on the "Victim Channel" and broadcast your fall while falling.
5. Doing a "Spiritual Bypass" through the lessons your fall is here to teach.
6. Living in the past and future—splitting into two while falling.
7. Trying to make the old you fit in with the new you after a fall.
8. Trying to become someone you are not so others cannot see you failing and falling.

9. Stacking fails on top of falls for an overwhelming fall.

10. Letting guilt be your destination instead of allowing your fall to just be an experience.

"GOOD" GRIEF

Elizabeth Kübler-Ross, in her 1969 book *On Death and Dying*, suggests there are five stages of grief: Denial, Anger, Bargaining, Depression, and Acceptance. Learning how to fall and grieve can help you understand and slow down enough to heal after a loss or fall. It is much like pulling weeds. If you grab and extract too quickly, you just end up grabbing the tops. You think you accomplished your mission, but when you turn your back, up they come again. You must be willing to use tools and grab with a better grip (on your situation), and then with a thorough pull, you'll remove the weeds, roots and all.

What does all of this have to do with a book on health? Failures, guilt, chaos left unhealed, bypassed, or left stuck, can form emotional patterns leading to emotional eating. Grieving often hurts, but good grieving can bring you unexpected gifts.

RISING IN SPRING

> "Sometimes it takes a good fall to really know where you stand."
>
> — Unknown

You may have guessed it by now—the Majestic Plate Spinner is me, and the Dancing Bear became my second husband. Unfortunately, after a divorce riddled with guilt, I did not know how to fall, which also meant I didn't know how to get back up. As a result, I went from a "dietitian on a mission" to "a dietitian with no ambition." I tried to resurrect the old me, but each time I did, I would fall again. Matthew 9:17 says, "Neither do people pour new wine into old wineskins. If they do, the skins will burst; the wine will run out and the wineskins will be ruined. No, they pour new wine into new wineskins, and both are preserved."

There it was. I had chosen a new life, but I was trying to bring my old life with me. I was trying to pick up all the broken pieces of plates and put them back together to look the way they once did, which was impossible. I was already different. The events alone made me different. My current husband and I could not bring our pasts into the marriage and force them onto each other; if we did, we would risk perishing. But we certainly tried. After failing and falling enough, we learned we had to build anew.

"The best education we can ever receive is from the University of Adversity. It's the only institute of learning that rewards us when we fall."

— Jason Versey

I began to make lemonade out of lemons and turned my mess into a message. Thankfully, I became more relatable. In the past, while handing you a menu, I had the university education but not the real life education. My level of thinking came from a "rulebook curriculum," which only works well in a perfect white picket fence world. Not until I ate a whole humble pie could I pour out enough compassion to teach from a whole new level of thinking. Ironically, I did not know true happiness until the whole pie was done. Like the prodigal daughter, I found such sweetness in the successes on the return. I began to believe in a power that is always there and as reliable as the sunset and sunrise.

THE SEPARATION

Have you ever felt like you are just existing but not really living—like something is missing? The passion for my career I had felt once upon a time was missing. At first, I believed being busy distracted me from seeing the full picture, and certainly, you don't know what you don't know. After falling in my own health, I needed a new vantage point so I could identify and release things that no longer served me. I wanted to carry on in my career, but like the ole adage "physician, heal thyself," I needed a whole lot of healing first. I desperately wanted to heal and forgive myself for "breaking up" my family, so I tried mindful and spiritual readings.

I began learning about healing from *A Course in Miracles*, which also led me to the audiobook *Secrets of the Immortal* by spiritual guru Gary Renard. Renard suggests you and I are spiritual beings having a human experience and our bodies serve our minds, not the other way around. My eyes widened as I pressed pause to let that sink in. My world as a dietitian was heavily focused on the body, on diseases and symptoms; it was completely the opposite of what he was saying.

Something about what Renard said resonated. I believed it had to be true; nothing else seemed to make sense. He went on to say, "If the body is ill, it must be that the mind was thinking with ill thoughts first, as the body will only respond to the way you command it with your mind."

As Renard spoke, I questioned myself. "If that's the case, then I brought on perimenopause with my mind?" *A Course in Miracles* says, "You cannot transfer what you have not learned." My curriculum did not teach the mind, body, spirit connection. Certainly not the spirit part. We had learned counseling skills but very little about the mind. We had learned about the brain too, but Renard was talking about something different.

My mind traveled through my forty years of traditional and nontraditional medicine. It was like being kissed by Prince Charming and rising from a deep slumber. I realized that my career had taught me only to a point. I thought I was making a difference, but I began to question the effectiveness of the teaching and the menus as I began to lose the passion.

Then, it was as though two scrolls appeared like ghosts from Christmas past in front of me. I could see the list of the pros and cons and commonalities between both types of medicine. I could see both traditional and nontraditional medicine created billion-dollar industries with pills and diets, but neither conquered the upward trend of disease. Although I felt fortunate to be educated in both forms of medicine, it felt like living between separating parents who do not speak to one another, leaving the patient to choose sides.

Usually, nontraditional medicine uses a holistic approach with open-minded, empowering ways to heal. On the other hand, there are inconsistencies and many diet restrictions. Traditional medicine is an absolute necessity, especially for acute situations. Diseases such as type

1 diabetes requires insulin—there is no alternative. And if you are having a heart attack, you need to get to the hospital, not your naturopath.

However, despite the flaws in either medical tradition, both can create dependencies on medications with the side effects and prices that come with them. In all fairness, both traditional and nontraditional medicine encourage healthy eating and activity in most cases. However, implementation of their advice is often the problem. Both types of medicine come with costs. Neither is innocent, and unfortunately, patients are left wondering who to trust.

All of this confusion over who to turn to can further escalate when media personalities jump in with their inconsistent claims, acting as though they have medical degrees. In any given magazine, one might find a success story that suggests we should cut out fat, then pick up another that encourages fat. Yet the articles are inconclusive and conveniently leave out the total calories consumed. If you do not know the whole story, you're left to fill in the gap.

BRIDGING THE GAP

Are you confused?

It's unfair. I wanted so badly to have both sides of medicine get along. I just didn't know how to do it. I was about to throw in the towel and retire at fifty, but I heard a whisper suggesting I was almost there in finding the answers. Having both types of medicine gave me an advantage, but it was my "failures" and my light dimming that allowed me to slow down and listen. Science, food chemistry, and understanding nutrients and disease taught me one side, while alternative medicine taught me the benefits of yoga, meditation, and supplements.

What I had to work on was empowering my desire to rise again. It dawned on me that empowerment and/or desire are the prerequisites to adhering to any program. That is where it starts—in the mind. Find a way to empowerment and therein lies the answer.

I vowed to find a way, a formula, and tools to bridge the gap between these two types of medicine to help empower you. As a result, this book is different from most. Plenty of books on diets have been written from both sides of medicine. If one side, one type of medicine, was all there was to it, though, wouldn't it be a done deal? You are about to walk across a bridge between old and new, nontraditional and traditional, to explore a new curriculum with a new formula—one that leads to freedom through empowerment.

THE DOMINO DIET FORMULA

In 2018, I was invited to Dallas, Texas, for a *DreamBuilder Live* conference with Mary Morrissey, owner of the Brave Thinking Institute. As this energetic, petite woman walked across the stage in her high heels, I noticed she had bright eyes like my grandmother's and a smile like my mother's. I instantly felt at home.

Mary talked about her struggles. I was all ears as she gave me someone to relate to. She told us about when she had been in the hospital with nephritis (kidney disease) and been told she only had months left to live. Mary had a six-month-old boy, so she desperately wanted to live. Then a nurse came to her bedside to pray with her, but in an unfamiliar way.

The nurse said to her. "Everything is created twice—first in thought and then form. The chair you are sitting in, the gown you are wearing, the bed you are laying in were all created in the mind first and then made into form."

The nurse did not discuss Mary's lab work or a renal diet. Instead, she taught Mary to use her mind to heal, and with that, Mary learned the power of her imagination. The nurse asked her to develop a vision filled with pictures of holding her son's hand walking into kindergarten, seeing him graduate from high school, and being in the front row at his wedding. Mary was able to use her mind, her vision filled with dreams, to override her belief in her illness. In her mind, she dialed up the desire to live with empowering dreams.

During the conference, Mary explained the power of the mind, starting with how you think. I knew about the power of the mind, but it is downplayed in many medical fields. Yet medications can only be approved for prescription after studies have been done with strict procedures that indirectly support the idea of the mind's power in healing. Medications are approved only after being found more effective than a placebo (usually a sugar pill). Studies have two or more groups of participants. One group receives the test medication and the other a placebo. Neither group knows which they are receiving.

Some in the placebo group, thinking they are taking the new medication, improve. This is called *The Placebo Effect*. It verifies that healing is possible with the power of the mind. Yet rather than use this power, traditional medicine tends to jump to prescription medications. Both sides seem to believe in the mind's ability to help heal the body. So, at the very least, why not suggest both—mind and medicine? Is the failure to do so due to lack of belief or a lack of understanding and education? Why is there more belief in a pill?

Mary described the underlining sequence of events leading to all results in what she called "The Results Formula." I sat at the edge of my seat, captivated, as she described how your thoughts create your results. For me, she built the bridge.

My passion returned; a messenger of health rose in me again. While I had focused on results in the past, I now learned to look at the events leading to those results as a domino effect! We need to look all the way back to the first domino in the row. I quickly did my best to combine my studies of traditional and nontraditional medicine with this concept, adding a new synergy to my holistic studies. I could see that if the mind created diseases, it could create solutions too.

I was so intrigued by what I had learned that I signed up for Mary's life coach certification program at the highest level. When I was certified, my treasure trove of learning became life coach meets dietitian meets alternative medicine practitioner to better serve you. I applied "The Results Formula" Mary Morrissey uses to all areas of life, including health, career, wealth, and relationships, and niched it within my focus on health and wellness, creating what I call....

THE DOMINO DIET FORMULA

Thoughts⇒ Breath⇒ Hormones⇒ Feelings⇒ Actions⇒ Results⇒ Freedom

Has this kind of experience happened to you? You watch a wellness documentary that motivates you to change, and you vow to start tomorrow, but by morning, the desire has waned? You woke on the wrong side of the bed, opened the fridge to the same old ingredients, and following your old routine, rushed to work. The problem is that you didn't stop to set up supports, so it *seems* easier to default to your familiar morning routine.

Achieving new results requires doing things differently, and that requires patience. Do you remember when you learned a new software program? Perhaps you were intrigued by the new program and how it would improve your efficiency. But then, perhaps, the learning curve was frustrating, causing you to question if the new software was worth it. Was it? What outdated software would you still be using if you hadn't tried something new?

The time you spend with this book learning new ways to achieve your new health goals will require new strategies too. The common temptation is to fast-track the process, looking for overnight success. That option does not work. Studies show that implementing small steps along the way produces better results. In fact, this is the reason for the reflections at the end of each chapter; they are designed to help you realign and design while helping you understand old patterns and the action steps to allow you to implement new understandings. Ask yourself if your old patterns are working and allow yourself to rewire and adjust to a new way. As my mother would say, "Do it right the first time, and you won't have to do it again."

One more thing—it saddens me to know roughly 80 percent of women are unhappy with their bodies and the percentage of men is close behind. Each chapter also contains a positive affirmation. I will discuss why they are effective later, but for now, know they help you create new ways to see yourself. As Wayne Dyer said, "If you change the way you look at things, the things you look at change."

Awareness alone may not change behavior, but combining it with taking steps and a "rinse and repeat" method leading to continuous improvement will. Are you ready to be your own success story?

> "We are what we repeatedly do. Excellence, then, is not an act, but a habit."
>
> — Aristotle

REFLECTIONS

1. Write about a time you fell and how you coped.

   _____

   _____

   _____

   _____

   _____

2. How do you rise from a fall? Can you think of a fall you experienced where something positive happened that would not have otherwise?

   _____

   _____

   _____

   _____

ACTION STEP

Write a letter to the person you are today about the lessons you have learned on your rise after falls, be it in health or otherwise. Write about the negative and positive experiences your journey has taught you to this point. What do you consider as successful results in your health and well-being? Write to the person you hope to be. What are you willing to let go of to grow toward your optimal well-being?

SUMMARY

At some point, everyone experiences shame, guilt, fear, hurt, anger, and the taste of humble pie. The saying goes: "Some people come into your life for a reason, a season, or a lifetime." Perhaps opportunities and failures come for a reason and a season too, and few things are here for a lifetime, especially failure. Take the time to heed the lessons those experiences are here to teach you. Grief is part of learning. That emotion is trying to get your attention and introduce something new in which to immerse yourself. Take time to grieve because therein an adventure awaits. Once you embrace the blessings in disguise, the failures may not seem like failures after all. Perhaps society had unrealistic expectations of you once again. Who created the definition of success and failure? Who is your judge and jury? You have access to a gentler approach in which alternative and traditional medicine are bridged using a formula based on using your inner healer, starting with your *mind*. Release old ways, embrace new ones, and aim toward healing rather than focusing on "flaws." It is time for self-empowerment so you can rise and create results you will love.

In the upcoming chapters, as we discuss *what to eat*, it may seem different from curriculum you are used to. You might expect to read first about nutrients and menus, but this time, these will appear later. Let's work first on empowering you to experience new results. Refer also to my website www.TheDominoDiet.com for tools such as The Domino Diet Workbook, The Domino Diet Journal/Food Journal, Calendar, affirmation cards, and more to help you deepen your journey to self-love and freedom.

AFFIRMATION

> "I may not be where I need to be, but I thank God I am not where I used to be."
>
> — Joyce Meyers

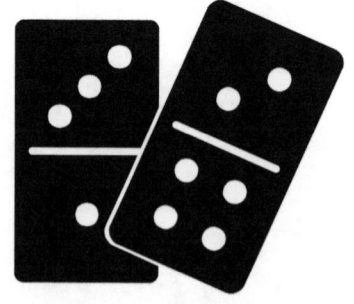

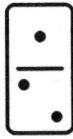

CHAPTER 3

UNDERSTANDING YOUR TWO MINDS

"When you rule your mind, you rule your world. When you choose your thoughts, you choose your results."

— Imelda Shanklin

Are you and I on the cusp of a new era? New eras begin with a changing mind where old ways are replaced with new, more efficient ones. The evolving mind never stops changing. Diets are in dire need of change. Is it time for new ways?

In 1967, eighteen-year-old Leroy graduated from high school. He dreamed of becoming a mechanic. His sixteen-year-old girlfriend Claire was still in high school and hoped for a career too. That year, however, changed the trajectory of their lives. An unexpected pregnancy meant Leroy and Claire would sacrifice their youth on behalf of another. The couple married and soon had a child to care for. Leroy struggled financially to support his new family; eventually, he was forced to look for work outside the area. He left his young family in his parents' care. His parents had their own financial struggles, so the most they could give him when he left was a sleeping bag, a spoon, and a can of beans. Leroy had to ration his can of beans for three days until he got hired as a janitor in a mechanic's shop.

Leroy's story starts like many—one minute you think you're going in one direction, but then life takes you in another. How you navigate your circumstances, though, makes all the difference.

While Leroy tended to his custodian duties, he watched the mechanics in admiration, still holding on to his dream of becoming one too. To make that dream become a reality meant picking up a second job as a door-to-door vacuum salesman so he could pay for training and to make ends meet. His vacuum sales boss recommended he read and listen to materials about how to boost sales. His boss knew the connection between an evolving mind and success. Leroy did boost his sales, and soon he had enough money to pay for his training and become a mechanic!

As a heavy-machinery mechanic, Leroy drove long hours to remote oil wells to service equipment. This time on the road allowed him to continue listening to and reading motivational materials. He was influenced by authors such as Wallace Wattles, Neville, and Napoleon Hill. By listening to these authors, overtime, Leroy's mind began to evolve.

The author Robert Collier, for example, studied the evolution of the mind after recovering from an illness using "mental healing." In his 1925 publication, *The Secret of the Ages*, he describes how the mind evolved and developed over time. For instance, the Stone Age was when fight-flight thinking was a necessary means of survival. The mind eventually created the Bronze and Iron Age when metals were used to enhance human strength and stamina. Eventually, the mind expanded to form synthetic items, including using metals to create our monetary system. Essentially, the mind changed from survival of the fittest to survival of the richest.

At the time of his book's publication, Collier said, "Now we are entering the Atomic Age, which is really the Age of the Mind—when every man can be his own master, when poverty and circumstance no longer hold power." Collier made that statement almost 100 years ago, but the power of the mind has yet to be used to the level he predicted, despite the possibilities and the inclusion of this same message 2,000 years ago in the Bible.

Catherine Ponder, author of the 1964 publication *The Prosperity Secrets of the Ages* wrote:

> You have the power within you, which you can use to experience greater health, happiness, and prosperity than you have previously known! You can begin releasing that power to produce greater good in your life and affairs when you realize that your mind is your world.

She, too, suggests knowing your mind and the power you hold can create abundance in all areas of your life. These authors point to mental development creating change.

Leroy's story demonstrates how, in a short time, the mind can evolve. In fact, his evolution continued. He honed his skills in sales and had a distinguished career selling the same machines he once serviced, winning national sales awards. His increased wealth became a true rags-to-riches story and one that will be clearer toward the end of this book.

This can all be attributed to an evolving mind.

Surely 100 years after the literature Leroy used was written, it is time to consider using the mind to improve our health. Do you believe the power of the mind can create a "wealth in health"? It starts with the mind and how you "mind your mind."

MINDING YOUR MIND

> "Your subconscious mind cannot argue controversially. Hence, if you give it wrong suggestions, it will accept them as true and proceed to bring them to pass as conditions, experiences, and events."
>
> — Joseph Murphy

It all starts with thoughts. The book you are holding, the chair you are sitting in, the walls in your home, and the electricity running through them are all energy that was formed by thoughts. Extending from your home, the trees, birds, galaxies…everything, including you, is energy. Some things vibrate at a higher frequency while others vibrate at a lower one, including your varying thoughts; even the thoughts you are unaware of. If you think positive thoughts, you emit positive energy and can create positive results. The same can be said for negative thoughts—spoken or otherwise—they all produce results.

Both science and religion have marveled over the power of the mind in various ways. For example, the Bible tells us "Believe that ye receive and ye shall receive" (Mark 11:24). Believing comes from the mind. The Bible also says, "Be ye transformed by the renewing of the mind"

(Romans 12:2). In other words, transformation or renewal also starts with the mind. In *The Power of Awareness*, Neville suggests, "Health, wealth, beauty, and genius are not created; they are only manifested by the arrangement of your mind."

It is safe to say the idea of the power of the mind goes back even farther than the century-old information Leroy used. What would Leroy and his family's fate have been if he had allowed himself to be a victim to his circumstances rather than be empowered with his evolving mind? Would his dream of being a mechanic have remained in 1967? Leroy minded his mind and used it to transform his situation for the better. What about today then? Do we still have power in our thoughts and minds? Let's stay *open-minded* and grow even more possibilities in our minds.

THINK AND GROW YOUR MIND

> "Just as our eyes need light in order to see, our minds need ideas in order to conceive."
>
> — Napoleon Hill, *Think and Grow Rich*

Have you ever been thinking of someone you rarely talk to when the phone rings and it's them? Or you're craving a cup of coffee from your favorite Java Junction when your friend shows up with a cup in hand?

You might recall the popular documentary, *The Secret*, that introduced many to the "Law of Attraction," but this law is actually preceded by the "Law of Vibration." Your thoughts have a vibration and can attract and/or create things on the same frequency. On a biological level, your thoughts communicate a signal to your corpus callosum, located between the right and left hemispheres of your brain. The corpus callosum then sends an electrical pulse, transmitting signals through the fluid running through your nervous, cellular, and molecular systems. Therefore, technically, your thoughts directly impact your entire body on an energy level. Think of an embarrassing thought and your cheeks flush, all from a thought. Whether the thought is in the past or the future, you still produce the same chemicals in your body as though it is currently happening. Recall a time you fell in love and you can instantly generate a similar response in your body.

Complaining or gossiping, be it in your mind or out loud, produces a corresponding inner chemical reaction where you bear the brunt of these thoughts, good or bad. In *As A Man Thinketh*, James Allen wrote, "The body is a servant of the mind. Disease and health, like any circumstances, are rooted in thought. Sickly thoughts will express themselves through a sickly body." In other words, you are using the Law of Attraction and/or Vibration to manifest health or sickness.

If one thought can alter your body chemistry, what about repetitive thoughts and their correlation to disease or health in the body? Wallace Wattles, in *The Science of Getting Well*, said, "You have a mind-body and a physical body; the mind-body takes form just as you think of yourself, and any thought which you hold continuously is made visible by the transformation of the physical body into its image." If everyone fully understood this, our minds would all act like the guards at Buckingham Palace to ensure no negative thoughts entered our minds. Instead, our belief in pain and medications has given us collective amnesia that blocks out this eternal wisdom. Based on Wattles' knowledge, once again we can conclude that if you want health, focus on health rather than disease. You cannot think on one frequency and produce results on another. Sickness and health are on different frequencies.

> "As someone thinks within himself, so he is."
>
> — Proverbs 23:7

The impulse to think about sickness is not entirely your fault. A whole industry has been built on sickness. Turn on the TV and you are bombarded by an onslaught of prescription medications and disclaimers describing even more forms of sickness with their corresponding side effects. Who benefits if you think more about sickness than health?

The good news is that thinking about health produces more health. As the saying goes, "Energy flows where your attention goes." Where does your attention go? Raymond Holliwell, a revered author in the world of Transcendentalism, wrote in *Working with the Laws*, "If you want success in living life, you must exercise intelligent discrimination of your thoughts." Choose healthy thoughts….

YOUR TWO MINDS

> "Disease is the result of a cause unconsciously established in the subconscious mind of the person ill. Where there is order and balance at the subconscious level, health will be obvious in the body."
>
> — Raymond Charles Barker

Let me state upfront that I am no expert in the field of the mind. Plus, a plethora of books on the mind have already been published. I do believe, though, that a gap exists between using the power of the mind in health programs and how the mind works for and against health. The complexity requires some exploring, which we will do throughout this book. First, let's start with your two minds and their extreme power.

The Subconscious Mind: The subconscious mind makes up about 90-95 percent of your mind and runs on autopilot, keeping your vital systems, such as your heart, lungs, and digestion, functioning. If it were not for this system, you would have to make yourself think and breathe every breath and beat every heartbeat, and so on. Your subconscious mind responds to all thoughts, be they positive, negative, unnoticed, or imagined, and treats each of them as though they were real. It also tracks and records every single thought and experience.

Since birth, your subconscious has been learning and recording events, emotions, and behaviors. Every movie you have watched, the color of the room you were born in, your emotions, etc. are all stored. Your subconscious is very literal and without a filter, which is best since it doesn't just decide to keep some things and throw away others. This is extremely important because otherwise it might make decisions like taking a rest from breathing when you are tired. Being literal, it does not have the capacity to determine what is worthy, just as a computer with uploaded data you provide can't distinguish between whether you are joking or being sarcastic or serious; it just uploads what you ask it to—all of it.

As stated earlier, everything begins with a thought. The job of the subconscious mind is to automatically give what you are thinking about form, directly or indirectly. If you say, "I feel tired," it will go to work finding ways to create tiredness for you. If you say, "I'm coming down with a cold," it will find a way to deliver that too. Fortunately, it works the same for positive thoughts, and the more you think those positive thoughts, the more positive habits form. This is the reason affirmations like "I am in perfect health harmony" are effective and why they are included at the end of each chapter. Like a genie in a bottle, your wish is your subconscious mind's command.

Herein lies the challenge because you are always thinking and often inconsistently. One minute you might be dreaming about a beautiful vacation and the next worrying about the money to pay for it. Even thoughts in your awareness can oscillate from *I should go for a walk* to *I feel too tired to walk*. Meanwhile, your subconscious oscillates to deliver results wherever you place your attention the most. If you are unhappy with your results, reassess your thinking. Are your thoughts clear and specific? If you think, *I want a lot of money*, your subconscious does not know what "a lot" means, and you cannot cash a check that says "a lot" of money. The same for goals such as "I will eat less sugar." There is no specificity, so your subconscious doesn't know what "less" means. The clearer, more precise, and consistent your thoughts, the better the chance of getting the results you want. In these examples, change to *I want ten thousand dollars* and *I will quit eating a candy bar every night*. Then your subconscious is clear on what you really want.

The Conscious Mind: The conscious mind comprises about 5-10 percent of your mind. It critically and logically examines your surroundings based on input from the five senses. Unlike the subconscious, it does filter, decipher, and make decisions. Think of your breathing right now. Your subconscious is controlling your breathing, but your conscious mind can change the rhythm of your breathing. The same can be said for your decision to eat for heart health. Your subconscious systems keeps your heart pumping. But you can choose to eat foods that improve your circulatory system. The key is how you make these choices. This will become clearer with in the *Domino Diet Formula*, which will weave through the following chapters. Understanding your mind can help you create a collaboration between your subconscious and conscious mind. It can also show you why willpower alone has not always been the best approach.

EMPOWER VS. WILLPOWER

"If we could get your subconscious mind to agree with your conscious mind about being happy, that's when your positive thoughts work."

— Bruce Lipton

Have your "two minds" argued about eating ice cream? Who's arguing and who decides? This is a gamechanger in my opinion. Simply saying, "I want to lose weight" doesn't usually work due to arguments between the minds. The decision to lose weight is made by the conscious 5-10 percent of your mind, but that can butt up against the subconscious 90-95 percent. Notice the percentage variation? Your body requires fuel to survive; therefore, skipping meals or eating restrictively can trigger your subconscious, which doesn't care about *Vanity* or *Vogue Magazine*. When you lose weight, the subconscious has no idea whether it was voluntary or due to illness and will seek to replace the weight and heal the body. Plus, when you lose something, your subconscious remembers, in most cases, you prefer to find what you lose. While I am simplifying the complexity of these "minds," the bottom line is that new strategies are needed to work with all the parts of the mind to increase the odds of success.

You are undoubtedly familiar with willpower, which uses your conscious mind but can feel like "force or push energy." Kirsten Welles, master coach with the Brave Thinking Institute, suggests, "The use of willpower alone is like holding a beach ball underwater; you can only do it for so long." Using willpower and its force energy to avoid eating ice cream often creates a sense of sacrifice. On the other hand, empowered thinking operates from a "lift energy." Empowering thoughts will sound more like *I enjoy ice cream with a quality over quantity mindset.* These thoughts come with a little more hope, a little more "lift energy," and less force.

Even more so, the "Will-to-Empower," using your subconscious and conscious mind in collaboration, can increase success. Learning to drive is an example of the use of both aspects of our mind, and after enough repetition, using the conscious and subconscious together becomes a habit. The desire to drive dials up the need for collaboration between conscious and subconscious and facilitates tolerance for the repetition. This programming occurs with learning to ride a bike, playing an instrument, or learning a new language, which are all learned by repetition. Keeping your desires and using affirmations while avoiding "all or nothing" thinking about goals will help your "minds" collaborate without setting off alarms. You will discover how going for a short walk can become a habit. They say, "Two heads are better than one." Well, "two minds" working together are too—even if they are in the same head.

HOW TO "HANDLE" YOUR THOUGHTS

You are always thinking; you are never not thinking. As all thoughts produce results, handling your thoughts can create better results. The trouble is your unnoticed results produce results too. When your mind is focused on an argument with your spouse or the throes of passion, you are on your way to results playing out in real-time. Using your conscious mind, you can notice your thoughts and determine which ones you want to keep before they produce results.

Start by looking at your current results. They will tell you what you've been thinking. Second, catching thoughts like, *I can't help it. I always crave chocolate,* can help you repattern them before you eat more chocolate. Always statements are almost never true anyway. Do you wake up craving chocolate? Try thinking and making empowering statements like, "I crave chocolate sometimes." Don't forget that your subconscious is listening and will deliver what you ask for in your thoughts.

Third, practice catching your thoughts. One strategy from Mary Morrissey is to notice your thoughts each time you touch a handle—door handles, drawer handles, faucet handles, etc.—and ask, "How am I handling my thoughts?" You will begin to see your thought patterns with this heightened awareness and strengthen what is called metacognition (self-thinking).

To provide an opportunity to repattern with more empowering thoughts, rather than saying, "I have to go for a walk," use affirmations like, "I enjoy how I feel after a walk." Which voice would you rather listen to?

> "Healing is a thought by which two minds perceive their oneness."
>
> — *A Course in Miracles*

FEEDING YOUR THOUGHTS

A youngster out walking noticed two dogs near their master. One dog seemed playful while the other was quite snarly. When the two dogs began fighting, the kid asked their master, "Which dog will win?" The master replied, "The one who was fed the most."

You have undoubtedly heard variations of this parable before about the thoughts you feed the most, the angry ones or the happy ones. To expand on this idea, did you know most, if not all, thoughts are either about the past or the future? If you experience anger, fear, or resentment, chances are your thoughts are mostly in the past. If you suffer from worry, panic, or anxiety, you may be anticipating or thinking about the future more. What thoughts do you feed the most?

Ironically, both patterns of thinking are illusions because the past no longer exists and the future hasn't happened yet. The only time that is real is the present moment. The present moment is the Holy Grail of thoughts. Have you ever had a headache, but when you got distracted for a moment, you suddenly forget about it? This relief is compliments of the present moment, where the truth resides. For example, you could be anticipating eating lasagna at lunch even when it is still breakfast. You aren't even hungry yet, but you are already deciding. You might even be deciding how much you will have since your past thinking is claiming you *always* overdo it with lasagna. In the present moment, when you are truly hungry, you can mindfully decide when to eat and when to stop.

More importantly, anxious or depressed thinking can go unrecognized, and as such, it leads to emotional eating.

How do you feed your thoughts, and which can you let go or grow?

> "Limitations live only in our minds. But if we use our imaginations, our possibilities become limitless."
>
> — Jamie Paolinetti

THE SCIENCE OF GROWING YOUR MIND

> "Every single blade of grass has an angel that bends over and whispers "grow, grow."
>
> — The Talmud

Do you want to improve your memory? Did you know you already have perfect memory? Under hypnosis, you can describe the day you were born, right down to the color of the room. Remember, your subconscious records everything. However, trauma, stress, and fear can cloud your memory. You are likely aware of how trauma can create amnesia as a protective mechanism to shield the mind from negative events. Did you know multitasking can also cloud your memory? Imagine you are eating your toast while heading out the door. You've set your keys down to let your dog in. You then run to your vehicle, and while gripping the toast between your teeth, you try to start your vehicle—but you forgot the keys on the counter. Is this caused by your poor and/or aging memory or distractions?

Memory loss is often blamed on age, but more is going on. Memory loss also coincides with less learning. Most learning takes place when we are young. In fact, in the first two years, your mind operates at a genius level, receiving constant stimulation. Later, once you have mastered so many things, learning dwindles. When learning new tasks, you use both your conscious and subconscious, and your brain is literally forming new connections (neural pathways), branching, and growing. If, however, you remain mostly on autopilot in your day-to-day routines, your growth is limited.

Can you do your job with your eyes closed? Before blaming age on memory loss, consider taking a course or learning an instrument. Even something as small as brushing your teeth with your opposite hand will engage your conscious and subconscious minds.

When you grow a garden, you know to add fertilizer for optimal growth. You can fertilize your mind's growth too. Studies suggest a healthy diet rich in vitamin E, fish oils, nuts, etc. can optimize brain health. Like your garden, sometimes a little weeding is needed too. Stress management is like weeding. The mental health benefits of meditating, uni-tasking, walking, hiking, yoga, etc. are extraordinary. Studies show that meditating as little as thirty minutes a day even while walking, for instance, not only helps manage stress but can increase mental acuity. A little food for thought.

FOOD FOR THOUGHT CRAVINGS

> "The greatest impediments to changes in our traditional roles seem to lie not in the visible world of conscious intent, but in the murky realm of the unconscious mind."
>
> — Augustus Y. Napier

If I say popcorn, you will not see the word popcorn; you will see an image of popped corn. That image is a thought. If you think of going to the movies, the association of popcorn might pop into your mind. Associations are thoughts too.

Cravings start with thoughts. Most believe cravings come from feelings. You have no idea what you will be feeling by the time you arrive at the movies, but your cravings are already being primed by your thoughts, not the other way around. At home, while watching TV, plenty of "food for thought" associations are brewing.

The point I am building to is that the chain reaction to cravings can begin long before the movies. Consider the influence of thoughts with the opposite of cravings like food aversions. Just the thought of some foods might make you cringe with nausea, dulling the appetite. Imagine slicing lemons and soon your salivary glands will react without a lemon anywhere near you, all from thought.

When you think of Christmas, what food associations come to mind? Do you crave shortbread cookies, eggnog, and candy canes throughout the year? Probably not, since you need to think of them first. Unless you think about Christmas all year long, I suspect you don't crave eggnog or shortbread all year long either.

Did the mere thought of cookies in this moment trigger cravings? Become aware of your thought patterns and you can conquer your cravings. They aren't as much a whim as many may assume. While feelings are involved, thoughts are first. If you just focus on feelings, you will miss the real culprit.

Have you heard, "I can't help it; I crave chips until they're gone"? Is this true? If you truly crave chips until they are gone, you would wake up craving them for breakfast. You need to think about them first before you crave them. Therefore, you are one thought away from being empowered to overcome your cravings!

Many use the tool "Positive Priming Thoughts" to get ahead of cravings. An example of priming thoughts I mentioned earlier was thinking about eating lasagna at lunch while you are still eating breakfast; in this case, you are deciding how hungry you will be later and installing a food craving. If you can catch this priming thought pattern, you can replace it with positive priming thoughts instead like, "I'll decide what I love when the time comes." Catching strong attachments to foods due to subconscious patterns such as pizza on Fridays is an effective way of breaking these habits. Deciding on the day, in the moment, allows new thoughts that can override your habitual cravings.

Last, notice your supper and evening snack thoughts on the way home. These may have even more sticking power due to: 1) tiredness, 2) reward associations, and 3) TV triggers. Consciously deciding to stop having evening snacks will require trudging through all the routine patterns-built courtesy of the subconscious. Again, affirmations and empowering thoughts can come to the rescue. Saying, "I will have a healthy snack," rather than using willpower alone not to have evening snacks will have better results. Snacks are now at an apex in calories. For many, they are the highest calorie intake in their day, every day! It isn't popcorn's fault or Christmas' fault. Enjoy your traditions, stuffing and all. Just make your food for thought with *mindful* thoughts.

DOMINO DIET MOMENTS

Mindless Thought⇒Craving⇒Every Day⇒Yearly⇒Mindless Eating⇒Weighty Results

Mindful Thought⇒Decide Wise⇒Enjoy Guilt-Free⇒Walk⇒Desired Results

REFLECTIONS

1. What are your food associations during the week/weekend or holidays?

   _____

   _____

   _____

2. Do you multitask? How does this effect your memory and/or eating and digestion?

   _____

   _____

   _____

ACTION STEP

Place sticky notes or elastic bands on door handles as reminders to ask, "How are you handling your thoughts?" Are you thinking about the future, the past, or the present moment? Become present and repattern with, "What would I love to create at this moment?" Feel empowered.

SUMMARY

You have a physical brain, and you have two minds. Your subconscious operates continuously, tracking every event and heartbeat so you don't consciously have to. This tracking is all part of survival. Using your conscious mind along with your subconscious, you can collaborate and empower each to create results you'll love while conquering cravings also. Build new patterns with affirmations and by learning new skills to *rewire and fire*. Like growth in your garden where fertilizer can nourish, your mind will nourish with nutrients to help your memory grow too. You hold within you a "genie" to think and sow. Handle your thoughts with positive present moments, a little food for your thoughts. Go easy; be patient. Habits aren't created by doing something once but by enough rinse and repeat to enforce them in your mind, so create good ones.

> "It is your conscious alone which makes you sick, and it is the establishing of order in the conscious which makes you well."
>
> — Raymond Charles Barker

AFFIRMATION

I have the *will-to-empower*, I am *powerful*, and I attract what I *love*.

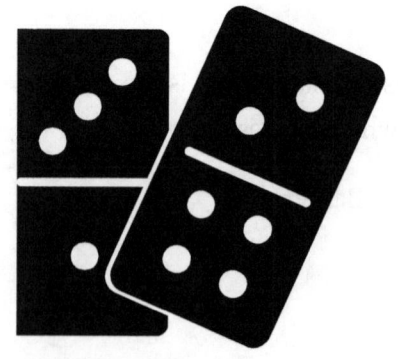

SECTION 2

THE SECOND DOMINO—EVERY LITTLE BREATH YOU TAKE

The Domino Diet Formula: Breath

Thoughts⇨**Breath**⇨Hormones⇨Feelings⇨Actions⇨Results⇨Freedom

---

You enter this world taking your first breath, and you leave this world taking your last. Scuba divers control their buoyancy, yogis meditate, and singers sing, all with breath control. How you breathe can bring panic or calm to the center of your being. You know that thinking makes it so; you are what you eat, but did you know you are how you breathe too?

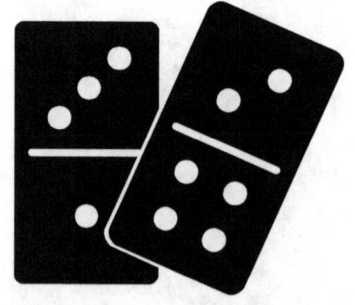

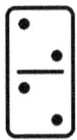

CHAPTER 4

TWO BROKEN HEARTS TOO YOUNG

"Breath is the bridge which connects life to consciousness, which unites your body to your thoughts. Whenever your mind becomes scattered, use your breath as a means to take hold of your mind again."

— Thich Nhat Hanh

I spent a portion of my career working in the intensive care unit (ICU) of a hospital. It is a place where quick, life-altering decisions are made. It is a place where survival mode thinking is in full bloom and where, "*Breathe*, everything will be okay," is a common phrase.

The ICU is filled with rushing energy, loud intercoms, beeping machines, zapping paddles, and exclamations like, "They stopped breathing!" It was my normal to be around watching the frontline staff. One day, though, something crept up from behind, nudged me, and said, "This is far from normal, nor should it be normal."

It was a Friday afternoon when Calvin scurried to the hospital with shooting pain down his arm. The intercom blared, "CODE BLUE!

CODE BLUE!" sending the white coats and scrubs running down the hall. It didn't matter what they had been doing—it was *go time*!

What was unusual to this particular scene was the thirty-two-year-old, six-foot, 185-pound male with no family history of heart disease who was diagnosed with a myocardial infarction (heart attack). This was the '90s when heart attacks stereotypically happened in older, overweight males. Although heart attacks were far from uncommon, they were unheard of in younger patients. Heart attacks were the number-one cause of death then, as they are today, but they correlated with the older, overweight male. Seeing a young, reasonably fit male diagnosed with a heart attack was a red flag in my book!

If that wasn't enough, another triage, code blue incident happened the same afternoon. Todd, also male, thirty-two, five-foot-ten-inches tall, and 178 pounds, was yet another atypical heart attack patient. The cases were not a week apart, not a day apart…they were an hour apart! That was the day the helter-skelter pace moved in slow motion for me. The cacophony of beeping monitors, IV drips, and intercoms swirled around me as my eyes spun slowly on a slow-motion merry-go-round. All I perceived were fires and staff running with extinguishers. I slowed down enough to ask, "Where are all these fires coming from, and why aren't we preventing them?"

I could feel a fire rising in me, knowing funding poured in on the sick but little was spent on preventing sickness. It was a hospital, after all, and already underfunded. On that day, though, the disparity struck me as odd. I knew there was so much that could be done to prevent illness, but the focus on fires kept the frontline staff running and completely exhausted. There was no time for holistic assessments, to ask patients about their stress or other potential culprits. I couldn't even do a full assessment of their diet. They were either incoherent or dealing with shock and their brush with the Grim Reaper. My job was to be ready to ensure nourishment with tube feeds or central line feedings, etc. By the time things settled, these two young men would be off to another unit for rehabilitation. To this day, I know very little about these two men who created in me a pivotal awareness—*prevention needs attention.*

Hospital funding was bleak and used to support an acute care model. Chronic diseases, such as heart disease or diabetes, were often treated using this acute care model. In the early 2000s, *chronic care models* began (in my awareness), but as you can well imagine, they are still in their infancy. How could years of solving both acute and chronic issues with one model suddenly have all the bugs worked out?

As often happens, fear can be behind the drive to include chronic care models. Fear lurks in both types of diagnosis. But fear alone does not guarantee long-term change. Studies show that within six months, fear often subsides, and life stresses reunite with old habits—pizza and wings for dinner on Friday. The motivation required to lower cholesterol, salt intake, and get off the couch is rarely sustained efficiently by a one-time message. Remember, in such cases, the 5 to 10 percent of the mind that is conscious is trying to argue with the subconscious 90 to 95 percent, which is accustomed to your usual lifestyle. One place to begin is to let go of fear-based thoughts and bring in another approach.

LETTING GO IN TRANSITION

My first experience of scuba diving was unforgettable to say the least. Practicing in the pool was one thing, but descending in the middle of the ocean clinging to the anchor line was another. I bobbed up and down with the rope while waves thrashed and splashed. My heart raced; my eyes bulged; I was in full panic mode. The dive master signaled to me, "Breathe…stay calm…breathe…."

I finally calmed down and made my seventy-foot dive into a whole new world. Leaving my full-time job with benefits and a pension plan felt similar. I held on with fear until I couldn't hold on any longer. The signals for me to work in preventative wellness became too strong to ignore.

I developed a private practice where a whole new world awaited me. It gave me time to make a better connection with patients and a better assessment of their needs—and understand fully how stress is like gasoline to the fire of disease. Healthy diets are beneficial, but changing lifestyles to match them can be difficult. What comes first, the chicken or the egg? Does stress ignite negative eating patterns, or is it the other way around? If stress comes first, which I believe it does, then what? It requires a different way of thinking and being.

The other situation I realized made it more difficult to change once you are diagnosed is that you are then left home alone trying to overhaul your life by changing your diet. This, in itself, compounds the stress. Often a vicious cycle of fear and stress grips you while you trudge through the plethora of quick fixes and temptations. Deep down, you want to change, but confusion and stress can leave you wondering where to turn. At the very least, it is time to let go of fear tactics and forced changes. To properly heal would mean to slow down, manage stress, and breathe. Let go of stress and being swayed by public opinion and make stress management an important part of your healing—then you will discover that a new way and a whole new world awaits.

HEALING BREATHING

"Breath is the link between mind and body."

— Dan Brule

Courtesy of the subconscious mind, you are always breathing automatically. How you breathe, though, can involve your conscious mind. You can survive for a time without food or water, but oxygen is a moment-to-moment requirement. Deep inhalation for more oxygen and exhalation for optimal carbon dioxide exhaust is rarely explored to determine the magnitude of its healing power.

For centuries, Eastern medicine used breathing methods such as meditation, yoga, Pilates, and tai chi for stress relief and healing. Seanna Quinn, certified yoga instructor and wellness coach, suggests yoga and other breathing techniques connect your mind, body, and spirit and can enhance your immune system, reduce stress, and act as a prescription for lowering anxiety.

Quinn is not alone. Others like Kirsten Welles of the Brave Thinking Institute also describe conscious breathing as a way to center the mind, spirit, and body. The word spirit, incidentally, comes from the Latin word *spiritus*, which means spirit or breath. See the connection?

Heart disease is the number-one cause of death in First World countries, and studies suggest stress is a contributor. Could there be more done in the way of mind, body, and spirit stress management for those like Calvin and Todd as a preventative approach? I wanted to be able to incorporate these and the Eastern medicine practices, but I found myself saying The Serenity Prayer: "God, grant me the serenity to accept the things I cannot change, the courage to change the things I can, and the wisdom to know the difference." I needed new tools, and I needed new thinking. As John Boggs, CEO of the Brave Thinking Institute, said, "In order to obtain the results you do not currently have, you need to be a match in thinking for the results you want."

After almost thirty years as a dietitian, becoming a certified life coach gave me the tools I needed to treat the whole patient. How you breathe happened to be in the sequence of events in the results formula. If an acute episode of anxiety and even something as extreme as a heart attack can benefit from calm breathing, how might it affect your day-to-day practices? Calm breathing is a centuries-old technique, an inexpensive option with no side effects.

> "The mind is the king of the senses, but
> the breath is the king of the mind."
>
> — Hartha Yoga Pradipika

"WEIGHTING" TO EXHALE

In some cases, part of vital dynamic health might involve weight release. When you release weight, where does it go? While a portion of your weight is released as water, did you know that when you lose weight, the majority is lost through your breath as carbon dioxide (CO_2)? When you consume excess carbohydrates and protein, it is stored as fat called *triglycerides*. Releasing this fat requires a process called oxidation. James McIntosh from the University of New South Wales, Australia, suggests when ten kilograms of fat is oxidized, 8.4 grams will be converted to CO_2. He said, "These findings suggest the lungs are the main excretory organ for weight loss." Since you exhale about 17,000 to 23,000 breaths per day, this fact is worth a little exploration. With one hour alone of moderate jogging, you can increase your breathing seven-fold. According to many studies, conditions like sleep apnea and insomnia often correlate with weight gain.

While jogging may not be for some, Eastern medicine's breathing practices can also increase this respiratory exchange system and may be one of the reasons those who meditate and practice yoga also notice weight release. We need to rethink breezing past the significance of these therapies for a quick fix with medication and probable side effects that leave us at risk.

YOU TAKE MY BREATH AWAY

As mentioned previously, the definition of health includes clean, fresh air. Does your workplace or home have poor air quality and/or require you to wear a mask? Do you have lifestyle habits obstructing your breathing? In either case, wearing a mask or smoking, for instance, can cause fluctuations in CO_2 and accumulation of carbon monoxide (CO), causing potential headaches, irritability, anxiety, skin disorders, etc.

I have been privileged to watch several *smudge and pipe* ceremonies in which smoke and tobacco offerings are part of the ritual. I spoke with many elders who explained their centuries-old traditions using natural tobacco on special occasions. However, added impurities due to commercialization and chronic daily use have altered tobacco's original sacredness. Ironically, smokers often think cigarettes are relaxing when it is much more likely the associated routine of inhaling and exhaling provides the relaxation. Chronic inhalation of either cannabis or tobacco has also become common for many people as a form of "relaxation."

Cannabis has been around for centuries and was also used for celebrations and ceremonies. Some studies indicate cannabis may have medicinal benefits. Overall, considering a risk-benefit ratio, case-by-case scenario, and use of smokeless forms may be prudent, especially for those who have other breathing impediments.

The deeper you inhale either substance, the more CO goes into your lungs. In turn, the benefits of deep breathing are undercut by the altered O_2, CO_2, and CO ratios. Equally noteworthy is the effect smoke inhalation has on the elasticity in blood vessels. The increased constriction and contraction of vessels alters blood flow through the entire body and brings on a risk of a whole host of concerns like heart disease, high blood pressure, and memory loss. All of these are inherent risks when tampering with your pulmonary and circulatory systems.

Overall, if your situation requires a mask that takes your breath away, consider offsetting exposure with longer periods of walking, meditating, yoga, etc. The benefits of enhancing and/or purifying your respiratory system are priceless and inexhaustibly available to you.

THE DOMINO DIET MOMENT

Thought⇒Hindered Breath⇒Lower O_2/CO_2⇒ Less Sleep⇒Weight Gain⇒Disease

Thought⇒Deep Breath⇒More O_2/CO_2⇒More Sleep⇒Low Triglyceride⇒Weight loss

> "Breathe, darling. This is just a chapter. It's not your whole story."
> — S. C. Lourie

REFLECTIONS

1. Are you running on adrenaline? Are you exhausted at the end of the day? Describe your normal breathing patterns.

   _____

   _____

   _____

   _____

2. Think of a time you felt panic or extreme anxiety. What were the steps or tools you used to calm yourself?

   _____

   _____

   _____

   _____

ACTION STEP

Take a twenty-minute walk or meditate while focusing on your breath. While using calm breathing, think of a challenge or a body ache. Notice how the oxygen increase in your circulation is improving your symptoms as you generate more energy and think creatively to help solve your challenge. Also note your sleep patterns after walking, meditating, yoga, or calm breathing before sleep.

SUMMARY

Your thoughts signal your nervous system to activate a breathing rhythm. Whether in acute or chronic care, calm breathing is one of the first tools for transitioning from dis-ease to ease. In chronic disease management, breathing techniques to manage stress are worth consideration. Bringing back these simple breathing practices might be as significant as the discovery of the "Dead Sea Scrolls," which rolled back time. Let's roll back time and bring back the early remedies of Eastern medicine while bridging it with Western medicine. What if both practices worked together? Would that be the long-awaited answer to conquering disease? Perhaps with the combination of deep breathing (for more O_2 in and CO_2 out) and proper sleep, releasing weight can literally happen in your dreams too.

AFFIRMATION

I breathe with ease! I release that which does not serve and receive all that does!

Tip: For heartburn/acid reflux, calm breathing before eating and walking after meals can help with digestion. You can also try plugging your nose and closing your mouth; then exhale and blow; this will close the pressure valve at the bottom of your esophagus. If you are familiar with scuba diving, this is a procedure called "equalizing" that pushes the air out of your diaphragm to release pressure.

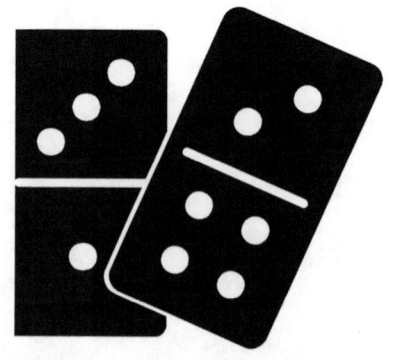

SECTION 3

THE THIRD DOMINO— HORMONALLY SPEAKING

The Domino Diet Formula: Hormones

Thoughts⇨ Breath⇨ **Hormones**⇨ Feelings⇨ Actions ⇨Results⇨Freedom

---

In the Domino Diet Formula, the third domino to fall is the one most widely misunderstood. This is where results begin to form in the body. From your mind to the way you breathe, you begin to create internal chemistry, and therefore, internal results. Knowing this formula can give you the awareness to catch potential "fires" before they spread.

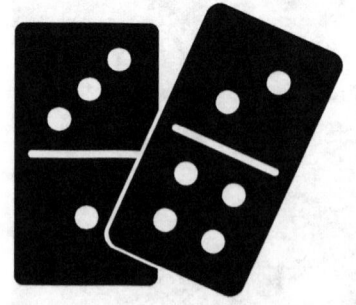

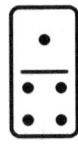

CHAPTER 5

SWITCH INTO THRIVE

> "Everyone thinks of changing the world, but no one thinks of changing himself."
>
> — Leo Tolstoy

Are your hormones out of balance? Do men experience menopause? When are hormonal changes normal instead of a sign you are out of balance?

Your feelings follow your hormones, yet most people believe it is the other way around. By the time you feel anger or cry tears, your hormones have already been working behind the scenes. Before you utter, "I feel calm" or "I feel anxious," a precursor happened to create your feelings. Once again, it starts with your thoughts, which dictate your breathing, which then signals your hormones. Feelings are the byproducts of your hormonal response. Therefore, feelings come after. If you are an emotional eater, exploring your feelings might seem logical, but it doesn't start or stop there. It goes deeper, as do the emotional battles with food.

Billy "The Kid," as he was often referred to, was told, "You look just like your father." Although he felt honored to look like his handsome father, it was a bit ominous—the last thing he wanted was his father's weight battles. Billy's father was morbidly obese, and Billy vowed to be different. Billy also dreamed of being an athlete. These two factors caused Billy to be active in sports. However, Billy also had his father's ferocious appetite. After gorging himself, he felt tremendous regret. By age thirteen, at the peak of his growth, his appetite was growing with him. Following the usual progression of growing teens, he gained weight, grew taller, then thinned again. His weight would distribute with his new height—until his height peaked. When his weight increased again, he was self-conscious but reluctant to talk to his father about it from fear of offending him. He didn't realize some of the weight gain was representative of his height, bone density, and muscle (which I will discuss more in an upcoming chapter). Fearing the worst, he decided to cut back on meals and increase his activity. It was easy for him to hide how little he was eating due to his parents' busy schedules. However, Billy's coach noticed a change in Billy's strength and stamina and his reluctance to do the swimming portion of his training. Billy was on the verge of an eating disorder; at the very least, he had "disordered eating behaviors." His dreams of becoming an athlete were at risk. He didn't know his body was mildly malnourished, and like many who have dangerously restrictive eating habits, his hormones bore the brunt.

Leslie Beck, dietitian and author of *The Complete Nutrition Guide for Women*, has stated, "Girls as young as nine years of age become preoccupied with their weight." Girls are at risk of amenorrhea (delayed or stopped menstruation) from extreme dieting. In other words, while hormonal changes are normal in teens, some changes are abornormal, brought on by inefficient fueling. For boys, less growth and muscle development, and in girls menstrual cycle changes, can be an indicator. This problem doesn't stop with adolescence; it applies to adults also.

Without sufficient calories, the body deems certain functions as unviable. For instance, if the environment is unsafe for fetal growth, estrogen levels often go down, stopping menstruation and causing infertility. Depending on the severity, the Female Triad Syndrome can occur, which presents as: 1) Lowering metabolism by lowering hormones like estrogen, 2) Lower estrogen, increased risk for osteoporosis, 3) Lower estrogen causing low fertility. Your metabolism is designed for survival. When calorie intake is altered or restricted, the energy you consume is directed to your vital organs. All other systems are secondary. If you attempt to chisel your six-pack abs by cutting too many calories, it will likely be counterproductive because the body's protective measures insulate your core, where your vital organs are, depriving your muscles of needed nutrients. This is yet another reason restrictive diets may negatively affect fertility.

DISORDERED EATING

Growing children often have higher calorie and nutrient requirements. Without adequate nourishment, immune systems, growth, and even mental health are in jeopardy. Adults, although fully grown, still require nourishment for energy and functioning internal systems. No matter what your age, your metabolism is only self-sufficient to a degree. Like any other living organism, it requires water and food to survive. When your core systems (heart, lung, digestion) are restricted, everything else takes a back seat. Symptoms like headaches, fatigue, and frequent colds are prevalent because your energy is diverted to your core. A healthy immune system is needed for survival, but your metabolism will prioritize pumping your heart and inflating your lungs before any other hormonal responses. With all your internal function needs, you can well imagine that losing weight isn't a priority for your body, over your survival. As your hormones do their job navigating and balancing your intake and your internal needs, they are often blamed for being out of balance. Saying, "I have a low metabolism" or "My hormones are out of balance" is pointing in the wrong direction. Your perfectly orchestrated system may not be to blame. Who is the conductor of this orchestra? Internal harmony (balance) cannot be achieved in isolation. In fact, no harmony can be achieved alone.

Your body operates continuously under what is called your basal metabolic rate (BMR). On average, women have a BMR of about 1,400 calories a day, while men require an average of 1,700 or more. At rest! To have optimal well-being requires optimal nourishment. Yet most fad diets total about 1,200 calories a day. This can ignite risks and alert hormones to adjust accordingly, which hormones are then blamed for. Any detected threat will signal all systems to preserve energy and slow your metabolism. Of course, this comes in handy if you are stranded on a desert island, but that situation is highly unlikely. Meanwhile, your BMR subconscious system packs more power than your efforts to release weight. Using your conscious mind cleverly, though, you can figure out a slow, steady, and less chaotic restrictive regime. There is a fine line between disordered eating and eating disorders. Understanding your body, monitoring signs indicating your hormones are making adjustments, and knowing they are alerting you is one place to start. Pay attention to clues such as tiredness, headaches, dizziness, frequent illness, lower strength/stamina, and weight plateaus. Weight plateaus incidentally tend to occur after fairly rapid weight loss when there seems to be a halt in losses. In upcoming chapters, I'll discuss strategies to help release weight with less hormone upheaval. For now, the focus is on your hormones and you as their conductor, not the other way around.

TAKING FLIGHT

Part of your survival is credited to your extremely well-orchestrated *sympathetic nervous system*, home of the fight, flight, or freeze response. For simplicity, I will refer to this as the "fight-flight" response. In the past, this system helped us run from predators. Big or small threats—animal or spouse, tyrant or traffic—the same response quickly kicks in today. We can be thankful for this instinct. Without it, humankind might not even be here. And we still need to use it, like in the ICU when the need for quick life and death decisions is ever present. However, the odds of needing to flee a mammoth, save a life, or freeze as I did on my scuba descent are less and less likely today. Still, the tendency is for the body to react with the fight-flight default even while driving in slow-moving traffic while in a hurry or arguing with someone. Any situation can trigger a response causing a flood of corresponding hormones—just like you're under attack—and some of these stressors are present every day.

Under stress, the brain receives a signal generated by your breathing and switches on all "needed" mechanisms. When the fight-flight response is triggered, your heart rate swiftly elevates and you release stored sugar (called glycogen) from your liver to fuel your muscles. Even your digestion wanes as your body focuses energy on stamina. However, if your stress response happens while driving, chances are you are not using your now well-stocked muscles to flee. Later, your system will crave food to restock your glycogen supply that was released from your liver even if it wasn't used by your muscles. And if you are under stress daily, your system simply does its job and asks for fuel to prepare for the stress response again and again. Further, imagine eating while driving or watching a horror movie—what is your heart rate doing? Remember, whether it's big or small, you could be having a stress response. If you can maintain your calm and cool while speeding, eating, and digesting, you are unique. Your conscious mind needs to be in overdrive to constantly keep tabs on the subconscious. This is certainly a worthy note for those struggling with anxiety and panic attacks.

Do you have digestive disorders? How well are you absorbing and digesting? Do you see the connection? Multitasking, driving, or being in any stressful situation increases the fight-flight response while you eat. Not only does your body slow digestion under this response, but you risk being supplied with more glycogen. Then your pancreas will produce even more insulin output than it did in the first place. There is nothing wrong with insulin—you need it to survive—but it is a fat-storing hormone. Moreover, one of the major hormones involved in stress is cortisol. Cortisol is also a fat-storing hormone. Consequently, you are eating your sandwich in a less than optimal digestive environment with added fat-storing enhancers. Your hormones are only trying to help steer within the environment you create. Meanwhile, bread is blamed for weight gain or digestive concerns.

HELPFUL HORMONES

You have more than fifty hormones, each of which is assigned its own unique role. They respond like well-trained troops ready to help as they were programmed. Once again, your mind triggers a breathing cadence and signals your hormone troops to respond. Your hormones don't decide on their own—your mind is in charge. Once your hormones are enlisted, a chemical reaction happens. For instance, the fight-flight hormonal response signals your heart to beat faster, supplying more blood flow, and your eyes widen to scan your environment. This all stems from your instantaneous thought. I am emphasizing this because we tend to blame the body, which is backward. Blaming emotional eating on your hormones or feelings leaves the true landmines unexploded and you tiptoeing around them. You can, however, become a master at switching and disarming the fight-flight primal response by using your conscious mind and enlisting another cascading response.

DNA DECODING

The time has come. It is a new era. It is time to shift to newer ways. You have access to a master switch that will allow you to shift from the fight-flight response default to a different, pristine system—the *parasympathetic system*, otherwise known as the "rest, create, digest response." For simplicity's sake, I will refer to this system as the rest and repair or R&R system. The R&R system is also extremely well-designed, but it offers entirely different results. Calm, deep breathing engages the R&R, producing pleasure hormones such as serotonin, dopamine, and oxytocin. As the name indicates, rest and digestion happen by design, allowing optimal nutritional absorption and making you feel full. Also, the R&R response offers rest and healing with better sleep and may offer enhanced creativity too.

Both the fight-flight and R&R responses were passed down through the generations in DNA and altered by subconscious adaptations. Perhaps it is safe to say that your grandparents and their grandparents used the fight-flight to a larger degree in gathering and rationing food.

Hunting and gathering skills provided them ways to feed twelve kids, operating under daily survival from lack and competition compared to the abundance of a store on every corner. There was little time for "rest, digest, and create." You and I, however, are new to abundant supplies and safety; therefore, we are susceptible to marketing tactics persuading us to buy two for one bags of chips. After succumbing to their lure, we bring them home to a well-stocked pantry and with fewer mouths to feed. Today, rationing food is more about portion control. Our archaic survival needs are met and we have the ability and temptation to eat as much as we want. But we have new consequences too.

If you were told "eat what's on your plate" or felt the need to compete for food with siblings, you may still subconsciously carry this programming into your adulthood. Past conditioning may leave you feeling every meal is the last supper, wedging you into feast or famine thinking. When preparing dinner after work, do you cook in a flurry, rush to the table, and then compare your plate with everyone else's? You are hardwired to compete to survive; it is up to you to override this instinct. Abundance has not really been taught. How could it? Your grandparents and parents could not teach what they did not know.

But now you know, and you are a trendsetter. You have within you the ability to reprogram and recode.

NO NEWS IS GOOD CHEWS

The good news is you have a choice. You can decide to switch off the panic, the competition, and "rest and digest." Your ancestors worked hard paving the way for you, and as a result, you have more leisure time, relatively speaking. Unfortunately, by and large, it is filled with a screen. Even meals are spent watching screens. I could talk about how this affects socialization and your well-being, but right now I am addressing how screen-time releases health-concerning hormones and disease while eating. First, if your mind is in two places at once, it lends to mindless eating. The goal is mindful eating. Many who eat in front of a screen report a sense of incompletion and/or skip feeling full and eat more. Multitasking while eating not only can leave you searching for more later, but induce digestive issues. Often overlooked, but perhaps even more important, is what you do while eating. Do you watch the news? How are you breathing? Is fight-flight underway while you digest, while you internally are under "attack"?

The good news is when you consciously calm yourself and breathe in slowly through your nose and out through your mouth—like blowing through a straw—roughly three times, you initiate your R&R system. This rhythm signals the brain that you are safe since calm breathing is not typical when being attacked. The brain reads your breathing carefully and releases a subsequent cocktail of hormones. In this case, serotonin, dopamine, and oxytocin come to your R&R rescue. Below are the main hormones and their functions.

1. **Serotonin:** *Mood Stabilizer* activated by walking, resting, meditation, dance, and music
2. **Dopamine:** *Rewarder* activated by wins, self-care actives, eating
3. **Oxytocin:** *Lover* activated by being with pets, music, giving a gift, holding a baby

How you breathe in times of chaos, political upheaval, or struggle compared to holding a baby is vastly different. Become an observer of your thoughts and breathing while you *chew* and you can enhance digestion, nutrient absorption, immune function, and also feel more fulfilled. Even when your thoughts go unnoticed and anxiety arises, just breathe and repattern to good chews.

REPATTERNING

Science has long claimed that you and I only use a small percentage of our brains. If the brain continues to evolve, perhaps this will change too. Certainly, awareness itself, and the use of the conscious to repattern the subconscious, could be part of that expansion. Early humans were hunter-gatherers with amazing stamina and strength. This also meant sitting silently alone or in groups awaiting prey. Hyper-focused vision and attention ruled their thinking and allowed them to "bring home the bacon."

The honing of skills over thousands of years resulted in the majority of men and women being wired differently. Men have a heightened ability to focus on one task while using their compartmentalized brains as efficiently as possible. On average, they use 7,000 words a day, looking for quick solutions and the "bottom line" in situations, which is why they have an innate desire to quickly solve the problems of anyone with whom they interact. Men are ignited more by dopamine, enhanced by sex, sports, competition, and productivity. Women, on the other hand, have brains similar to a large ball of wire, giving them multitasking tendencies, and the ability to use about 20,000 words a day. Years back, they were tending to the fire, children, cooking, and gathering with other women, driven by oxytocin and heightened by feeling connected in conversations. However, their emotionally super-charged wiring makes them susceptible to feeling overwhelmed and anxious and to be "spinning" with thoughts.

It isn't your fault you are wired the way you are. Being aware, however, can help you repattern your thinking with your conscious mind. Think, for example, of how men and women could learn to manage stress by finding compromises through conversations and shared interests to reach a common goal. Why this really matters is it can otherwise trigger potential everyday stressors in relationships and lead to health problems. Could this also be why heart disease is the number-one cause of death today?

A woman who feels undervalued, unheard, or disconnected at work or home may crave oxytocin and/or serotonin and mistakenly attempt to meet the craving with chocolate instead. Men in the same situation might turn to action movies with snacks and "tune out the world" or hyper-focus on sex. Men are also more likely to turn to alcohol and substances for their erroneous dopamine fix. While there are distinctions in men and women's body chemistry, there are exceptions, and these DNA patterns may be altered through awareness. For example, connecting the dots of emotional eating can be the beginning of repatterning.

You cannot change something you are unaware of. There have been far too many decades of feeling flawed and pointing fingers. How can thousands of years suddenly change overnight? Time, patience, and knowing it wasn't your fault can take some of the pressure off. That, in itself, can help repattern your thinking, breathing, hormones, feelings, and your subsequent results. Your inner cave dweller is ready to transcend.

YOUR INNER CHILD, YOUR INNER BEAUTY

> "I'm happy to report that my inner child is still ageless."
>
> — James Broughton

Isn't it ironic that most couples see each other at the start and end of the day while tired and hungry? The world sees your beauty, but your partner sees your beast!

Hunger and lack of sleep are hormone-related too. Once upon a time, hearty late meals followed working laboriously in the fields, and occasionally, a light evening snack followed. Now, late evening meals and large snacks are the norm and the fields have been replaced by TV. Who doesn't love a "shut-down" at night? However, heavy, late snacks are digested through the night and into the morning, so now the trend is replacing nourishment when you wake. And the late snack has become one of, if not the highest calorie count in a day despite low-calorie expenditures. Unfortunately, heavy, late night snacks can cause: 1) sleep disruption and/or nightmares, 2) heartburn, 3) appetite fluctuations, 4) sugar and mood swings, and 5) headaches. Further, fatigue from lack of sleep can lead to less activity during the day. Alongside blood sugar swings, anxiety lurks and worsens with drinking more caffeine to stay awake—a compounding cyclical problem. The long and short of skipping meals, possibly leading to heavy snacks before bedtime and/or lack of sleep is a potential hormonal rollercoaster ride, and for some, it happens every day.

Sleep, disease management, and your appetite are all connected since sleep regulates specific hormones. Adults need about seven to nine hours of sleep per night. One study showed sleeping five-and-a-half hours per night while following a calorie-restricted diet produced less fat loss than for those who slept eight-and-a-half hours. The hormone *leptin*, responsible for increasing satiety, was higher in those with more sleep. On the other hand, the hormone *ghrelin* (the hunger hormone) increased the appetite in sleep-deprived subjects. Not only are you at risk of being a "Gremlin" when you're tired, but you might also be "hangry" more often. Sadly, far too many hours are spent tired and unfulfilled. What if love was there instead to soothe?

What if you had more energy during your leisure time rather than work consuming it all? It is possible with proper sleep and fuel. Whether you work regular hours or shiftwork hours, customizing the times of nourishing meals and snacks can help you have more productivity at work and help you arrive home with more energy to enjoy your precious leisure time too.

Suggested Meal and Snack Patterns

- Wake: "Break the Fast" (Breakfast) within **one hour.** If you struggle eating when waking, start small (yogurt, banana, or nut butter on toast) and eat light before sleep.
- Every **two to three hours**, fuel with small, frequent meals (three meals and two to three snacks per day).
- Not a "snacker"? Avoid going longer than **three to four hours** between meals.
- Have a small *snack* **two hours** before bed (optional).

Finally, sleep is often overlooked as a time for people of all ages to repair and recover. Children, for instance, produce more growth hormone during sleep. Plus, your immune system is at work while you rest and repair. Between 1 and 4 a.m., REM sleep occurs, and the hormones melatonin and serotonin further help you heal. Melatonin enhances sleep and is a rich antioxidant involved in cellular repair. Below is a prescription for "extra-strength" R&R to supplement your day and sleep!

R&R SUPPLEMENTS

- Spend time in nature.
- Get a massage.
- Pray, practice meditation.
- Breathe deeply (there are apps for that).
- Get adequate sleep.
- Listen to or play music.
- Be with animals.
- Walk, dance, do yoga or tai chi.
- Do crafts, art, or coloring.
- Write and/or cook.
- And more….

R&R Supplement Directions: Disclaimer—May cause increased creativity.

> "Breathe in slowly through your nose and out slowly through your mouth like blowing through a straw, at least three times in a row, make sure the inhalation and exhalation has a comfortable rhythm and pace for you. You can use this breathing practice as an 'energetic supplement' and take three times per day or as needed."
>
> — Kirsten Welles, Master Coach, Brave Thinking Institute

DOMINO DIET MOMENTS

Thought⇒Shallow Breath⇒Fight-Flight⇒Cortisol⇒Disease⇒Poor Sleep ⇒Disease

Thought⇒Deep Breath⇒Rest Repair⇒Serotonin⇒Ease⇒Sleep⇒ Health Harmony

REFLECTIONS

1. What is your default response? Fight-flight or R&R? Are your hunger and tiredness related, and if so, how can you fuel and adjust your routines?

   _____
   _____
   _____
   _____

2. Do you eat during screen time? How is your eating pace as a result? Does it cause mindless vs. mindful eating?

   _____
   _____
   _____
   _____

ACTION STEP

Create time in your day, such as at meals, to place yourself in the R&R system using the three deep inhales and exhales as discussed. Place sticky notes on your desk or table or use phone reminders. Try this three times a day and/or as needed.

SUMMARY

You have two well-orchestrated hormonal systems coded into your DNA. While "fight-flight" was your primary survival response, given the abundance in First World countries, protection, shelter, and food supply, perhaps the R&R system can become your default. Awareness—using your conscious mind to breathe and switch to rest, digest, repair, and create more often—might expand the mind and reduce disease. Although it is newer territory, as Leroy showed not so long ago when he lived on one can of beans for three days, your ancestors worked to pave a way for you. Imagine the sense of good fortune they would have felt if they had been able to fuel their day and rest with more leisure, doing what they love to do. You can do that because the anxiety and other side effects of the fight-flight response are in your hands and mind to control. Switch into R&R for optimal sleep, digestion, and ease away from disease. If you rise rested and arrive home energized, you might even have more love in your day by spending higher quality time with your loved ones. Your inner beauty will shine through too.

AFFIRMATION

I am surrounded by a perfect bubble of love and protection. I am calm, cool, and confident.

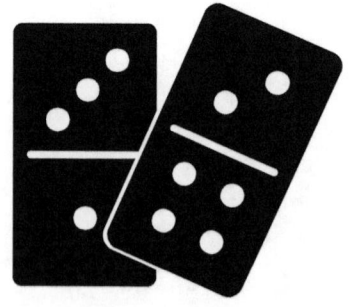

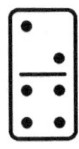

CHAPTER 6

MEN-O-PAUSE

"I'm still hot—it just comes in flashes now."

— Unknown

Kathy was the energetic one. She was always on the go and happily walking or running most days. Suddenly, around age forty, she started experiencing a series of ailments from bed spins (vertigo), pains in her lower stomach, hot flashes, thinning hair, weight gain, insomnia, and extreme fatigue. She tried to stay active and follow a low-calorie diet to stave off the unexplainable weight gain, but nothing seemed to help nor explain her symptoms. Finally, a trip to the doctor and lab work indicated irregular TSH, meaning her thyroid function was in question. In addition, low progesterone and estrogen pointed to a diagnosis of perimenopause at age forty.

Throughout their marriage, Kathy and her husband had been deeply in love and virtually inseparable. But when Kathy started to experience perimenopause, things took a turn. After a full year of hot flashes and dizziness, she was diagnosed with full-blown menopause. She was in

"Men-o-Pause" all right—her sex-drive drove away and left her with a spare tire around her waist. Kathy suggested going out for dinner to rev up the mood, but it also meant squeezing into Spanx and control tops to fit her wardrobe. Breathing was difficult, especially after a meal and a glass of wine, but wine gave her a flirtatious edge her husband eagerly awaited. However, the wine came with ten rounds of hot flashes. Arriving home, with her mid-section compressed like a twisted balloon, she finally undressed. Catching her reflection in the mirror revealed an hour-glass figure transformed into a substantial baby bump. Now, with melting makeup and bloated stomach, she felt more like she had just given birth. It wasn't Kathy's intention to go from feeling sexy to killing the mood. She wanted her youthful, fun, sexy side back, but her eyes filled with tears instead.

Meanwhile, after dinner, Kathy's husband, infused with wine that kicked in for him, had proceeded to pour on the charm, offering compliments despite her melting mascara and swollen red eyes. She couldn't recall hearing compliments while sitting in discomfort all night compressed in her dress. The difference between their moods now created tension in the bedroom. So many mixed emotions came with Kathy's changing hormones, compounded with the aging process. Kathy felt like there really ought to be a sign in her bedroom listing menopause survival tips. At the bottom in bold print it would say, "You aren't alone; I miss her too!"

MENOPAUSE

You have likely heard that once you hit menopause, it's harder to lose weight. While not all women experience the same symptoms in menopause, weight change seems to be the most common. However, it might also coincide with lowering activity—another domino effect in the wrong direction. A combination of less sleep, corresponding appetite changes caused by an increase in the hormone ghrelin, plus feeling depressed can alter calorie intake and expenditure. Feeling exhausted makes workouts more difficult. Hot flashes can indicate the fight-flight response is in effect, meaning cortisol levels may be rising too—a formula for weight change.

Menopause usually starts around forty-five to fifty years of age, when female ovaries stop producing estrogen and progesterone. After one year of consecutive missed cycles, you are considered menopausal. Many women experience hot flashes, insomnia, weight gain, lower bone density, lower sex drive, mood swings, joint pain, digestive problems, brain fog, and hair loss. Who wouldn't feel a little depressed? Seeing your body change before your eyes can cause grief. Hormone fluctuations can cause low blood sugar episodes, subsequent mood swings, and sensitivities to caffeine and alcohol as well as dehydration, which can also cause hot flashes and add to the looming depression.

In addition, consuming too much sugar can cause higher insulin levels, then cause low blood sugars, followed by an immense craving for more sugar and corresponding increased weight. A vicious cycle. There is hope, though, if you return to your thoughts; your conscious mind can create calm breathing and better sleeping, along with foods and eating patterns for appetite control.

On another positive note, studies show when women with polycystic ovarian disease or in menopause consume high fiber (low glycemic) diets, they may reduce insulin and blood sugar fluctuations. Lean protein combined with carbohydrates can also lessen blood sugar swings and calorie intakes. Studies also show consuming small, frequent meals can help manage heart disease, diabetes, and digestive diseases, all of which are higher risks in menopause. We will talk more about diet regimes in upcoming chapters.

HOT FLASH!

Besides weight gain, the other most common and noted nemesis of menopause is the notorious hot flashes! You'll know when you walk into the home of a "hot flasher" when you remain bundled in layers and she's wearing shorts with the heat off in winter. The battle between couples sounds like, "Well, you can always put a layer on. If I strip down anymore, it won't be PG!" The hot flash rollercoaster comes with an internal inferno eruption, insomnia from an increased anxious mind, damp sheets and restless legs, and exhaustion with a dampened desire to do the extra activity needed to fend off the involuntary weight gain. And this daily vicious cycle has an unknown expiration date. No wonder the cycle comes with a "Mood Bender" too.

Dehydration can create headaches, cramping, and dizziness, and spark even more hot flashes. As indicated earlier, caffeine and alcohol can exacerbate dehydration and elevate heart rates continuing the progression of hot flashes. It doesn't mean giving up coffee completely but monitoring your tolerance. A cup of coffee later in the day might have been fine at one time, but on behalf of your sleep hygiene, you may need a new cut-off time, such as Noon-2:00 p.m.

Good sleep hygiene is too often overlooked as is walking and/or meditation. Each of these allows the R&R systems to help offset the fight-flight reaction from catapulting you into hot flashes. Before bed, try smells of lavender and drinking chamomile tea. If you are prone to leg cramps, you may require potassium replacement foods due to frequent sweats. Incorporating high potassium foods (banana, potato, sweet potato, spinach, apricots, tomato sauce) or a low-calorie sports drink, especially in hot weather, can also be beneficial. Consider a small snack two hours before bed, such as a high fiber cereal or whole-grain toast with nut butter and half a banana to reduce symptoms.

During menopause, due to lowering estrogen, the risk of heart disease increases. Consuming red wine is linked to lowering heart disease by increasing good cholesterol (HDL), but consider the risk-benefit ratio. The national guidelines for women recommend consuming no more than one to two five-ounce glasses of wine a day. Depending on other risk factors, a glass of wine paired with a small snack, especially if you are prone to low blood sugar, is recommended. Surpassing these guidelines may offset the benefits and add to the risk of dehydration and hot flashes. Consider organic wines if sulfites ignite histamine effects, compounding hot flashes.

You have probably heard of adding one serving of soy products (tofu or soy milk) to help reduce hot flashes. It's worth trying. The emphasis is on one serving, once again, and if using soy milk, choose one fortified with vitamin D. Lowering estrogen can increase the risk of osteoporosis, so to increase bone density, include plenty of calcium and vitamin D in your diet, get lots of safe sun exposure, and do weight-bearing exercises. These can also have positive effects on mood stabilization.

Menopause isn't the same for every woman, but lower estrogen levels will be common for everyone, causing increased risk for other health concerns. Overall, it is best to increase your R&R response with walking, more sleep, hydration, less caffeine, lower salt intake, and less sugar while consuming healthy fats and foods high in potassium, fiber, calcium, and omegas. A glass of red wine in some cases and a serving of soy products is also worth considering, as is weight resistance training to stabilize hormones.

I would like to add that the herb *black cohosh* has been shown to help in some cases. Refer to my website (www.TheDominoDiet.com) for more specifics on diet and to see if adding supplements such as a women's multi-vitamin, added calcium, omegas, fiber, and added lean protein are advised.

Tips for better sleep: Sound machines, apps providing white noise, and a bedside fan all add up to a reasonably priced investment. Stay cool! If you think you have a sleep disorder, consider getting an assessment to rule out sleep apnea, etc.

*MAN*OPAUSE

Men do experience menopause or andropause. Generally, after forty, androgen and testosterone levels decrease. Symptoms can include diminished sex drive combined with episodes of erectile dysfunction. Often, men too have sleepless nights, fatigue, increased body fat, hair loss, and muscle loss. Whether it is the combination of these symptoms or a symptom of its own making, depression is more likely in men during this phase. Believe it or not, some men even experience hot flashes!

The good news is you can naturally increase testosterone with activities such as weightlifting. A diet high in zinc and vitamin D, and good sleep hygiene can also help. Of course, watching the waistline and eating smaller portions is important, especially since men have a higher risk of heart disease, particularly if they have an apple-shaped abdomen. Vital organs are held in the chest and abdominal cavity, and therefore, added adipose tissue (body fat) in this area can hinder organ functions. On top of this, excessive sitting, stress, weight increase, and specific foods can increase episodes of acid reflux. Although a glass of red wine can help with HDL cholesterol levels, consider the added calories from alcohol and the increased risk of reflux. Speak with your doctor and/or dietitian to help customize your diet. Overall, small, frequent meals, R&R, meditation, good sleep hygiene, stress management, walking, and weight training are great strategies.

A MIDLIFE AWAKENING IS NOT A CRISIS

It isn't about the red Corvette. Men overall have been given a bad rap for having what we call a *midlife crisis*. Is it a crisis to reach an age and wake up, realizing there is less time for things left undone or to wonder if there is more to give and receive from life? After sacrificing and putting your dreams on hold to raise a family, the kids move out and it is finally time for you to dream again. Instead, society sees it backward, embracing the working hard years until retirement instead of the awakening that awaits. To not awaken should be considered abnormal.

Unfortunately, the focus is on the "crisis," giving this stage of life a negative connotation. What if it was called an awakening? Whether it's traveling in a Winnebago or a red Corvette, you deserve rewards along your life journey. Maybe aging could be welcomed because we realize there is more after retirement, which would be an incentive to be in optimal health to enjoy it. How would you plan life knowing more dreams are waiting for you? What if more programs were dedicated to continued learning for people of all ages? Certainly, the conscious mind benefits as your memory expands.

What if hormone changes were seen through a compassionate lens of knowing there's more going on? In puberty, you say goodbye to your childhood. In adulthood, you say goodbye to your teens. In marriage and/or parenthood, you say goodbye to your individuality. In menopause/manopause, you say goodbye to childbearing and some vanity, stamina, and invincibility. As I mentioned earlier, Elizabeth Kübler-Ross, author of *On Death and Dying*, suggests there are five stages of grief when experiencing loss: 1) Denial, 2) Anger, 3) Bargaining, 4) Depression, 5) Acceptance.

Perhaps these five stages coincide with hormonal changes, but hormones shouldn't take all the blame. Each stage involves its own issues: Denial of age, wanting to be older, or wanting Botox to look younger; Anger based on vanity or a lack thereof; Bargaining and wishing for more; Depression over losing youthful qualities; finally, Acceptance, albeit wavering. What if there were compassion to grieve and support dreams? That is far from a crisis. Leave no stone unturned and leave the planet without regrets, knowing the fountain of youth is overrated. The fountain of wisdom earned you the Corvette in the first place!

> "There is the opponent that exists within each of us, and its sole purpose is to challenge us to overcome it, thereby becoming better versions of ourselves."
>
> — The Kabbalah

Tip: With hormonal changes and especially with hot flashes, you may notice more body odor due to dryness, urinary tract infections, and/or sweating. Stay hydrated, try clinical-grade deodorants, and for urinary infections, try concentrated cranberry juice.

DOMINO DIET MOMENTS

Thought⇒Fight-Flight⇒Disease⇒Hot Flashes⇒Less Sleep⇒Fatigue ⇒Weight Gain

Thought⇒R&R⇒Sleep Ease⇒Energy ⇒Active⇒Health Harmony⇒ Weight Managed

REFLECTIONS

1. Reflect on and explain past hormonal changes and your changing emotions. Was grief part of the changes?

   _____

   _____

   _____

   _____

2. Drawing upon what you just learned, list ways you can manage stress and/or symptoms of menopause/manopause.

   _____

   _____

   _____

   _____

ACTION STEP

Take a step toward your best sleep hygiene. Experiment with a cut off time for caffeine and nighttime snacks (snack size), allowing two- to three-hours for digestion. Try fresh air, a cooler room, and leaving a window open slightly. Consider a heated mattress pad with two zones to customize you and your partner's preferences.

SUMMARY

Hormonal changes have always been and will continue. Your hormones are doing their job preparing you for the next new phase of life. What we call a hormone imbalance is more likely a thinking and/or nourishment imbalance. The good news is you can build new, conscious habits. Allow yourself time to grieve and stay curious about the new you emerging from these natural changes. Make time for more R&R and to dust off an old dream or two. If you are compassionate and compromise amicably with your spouse, you can support each other as you change. No one is exempted from hormonal changes brought on by aging. Enjoy the Winnebago. Maybe it is pulling your red Corvette. With your fountain of wisdom, enjoy your mid-life awakening because it can help unleash your dreams.

> "Yes, I'm high maintenance but it's okay
> because I maintain myself."
>
> — Unknown

AFFIRMATION

I deserve a life I love living.

Tip: Create a vision board or create one on an app. Remember, your future growth and development does not need an expiration date. Get inspired. You have things left to do!

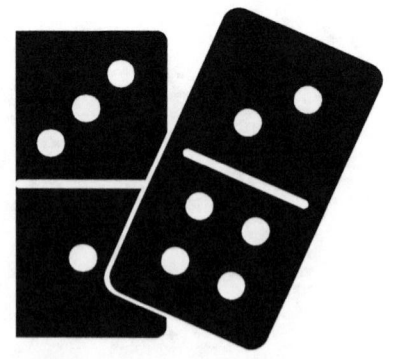

SECTION 4

THE FOURTH DOMINO—RISING ABOVE

The Domino Diet Formula: Feelings

Thoughts⇨ Breath⇨ Hormones⇨ **Feelings**⇨ Actions⇨ Results ⇨ Freedom

---

You have arrived at the middle of the Domino Formula. Good work.

In this section, we'll look at what happens if thoughts go unnoticed. Whether you notice or not, you still have a chance to change your results. Thoughts are the language of the mind, but feelings are the language of the body. Feelings and/or emotions have long been associated with emotional eating, but as you are now aware, they start with thoughts. The misconception of feelings dictating actions is due to it being an incomplete explanation. After all, feelings are in the middle of the formula.

Feelings are heavy influencers, but because they are the fourth domino in the chain reaction, they also can be repatterned with thought. Without awareness, the power emitted by feelings can either spring you into action or keep you stuck. The very reason diets tend to fail is thoughts and emotions either keep you trapped or pull you back into a trap even after you experience positive results.

Breaking free is possible, though, with tools to break the chains.

It might surprise you to know that fear and love might be holding you back under the name of self-sabotage.

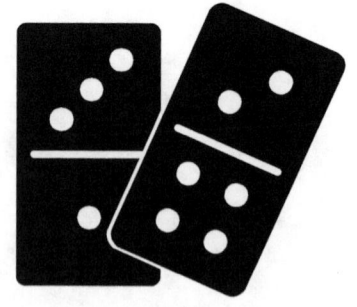

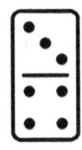

CHAPTER 7

DIGESTING YOUR FEELINGS WITH YOUR FRIEND JACK DANIELS

"Guilt is to the Spirit what pain is to the body."

— Elder David A. Bednar

Does a fight with your spouse, coworker, or teenager undermine your health? Is guilt, shame, or anger connected to disease and weight management?

Steve sat with his shoulders slumped, holding his burning stomach with one hand and his pounding head with the other. Sitting on the edge of his bed, it was all he could do to get up for work. The evidence of his symptoms and remorse was another empty bottle on the floor. The reflection in the mirror across from him was a man he no longer recognized. Thinning hair and reddened eyes with dark circles replaced his sparkling blue eyes and signature dimpled smile. The shame of a failed marriage and bankruptcy consumed him, as did the guilt of no longer living with his sons. He had moved to a dark basement with the clothes on his back and a suitcase in hand, and overnight, everything had changed. His boys were too young to understand and clung to their mother. Steve felt isolated and alone. It wasn't like it had been part of the plan or intentional to build a life and family and then leave. Was Steve having a midlife crisis or an awakening?

Prior to Steve's divorce, he was 300 pounds. He had been diagnosed with pre-diabetes, high blood pressure, and high cholesterol at age twenty-seven. His diagnosis and losing his mother were the first crisis that brought his awakening. It led to diet changes and workouts to the point of completing full marathons! In fact, he managed to lose a total of 100 pounds. However, his diet program did not come with coping skills, so he was unprepared when chaos came along again. As a result, he traded running for evenings with his old friend Jack Daniels. The willpower he once used against food and alcohol could not withstand his guilt and shame. It simply lacked the amperage to create change at the level of the mind where weight battles and addictions start. Trauma is multifaceted and arises to varying degrees, and it is a breeding ground for addictions and self-sabotage, demotivated energy, self-criticism, and being emotionally cut off. What diet can stand up to that?

TRAPPED AND TRIGGERED

> "All thoughts which have been emotionalized (given feelings) and mixed with faith, begin immediately to translate themselves into their physical equivalent."
>
> — Napoleon Hill

You aren't born with bad habits. They don't come with neon signs. They're seductively convincing and develop slowly like wrinkles on your skin and grey hair on your head. Steve was used to arriving home after work to excited kids. Then he went from a family home to a lonely basement unit. Driving home to his new makeshift home meant seeing images of sitting alone. He didn't plan to create an addictive habit. He thought, *I'll just grab one for the weekend* as he swerved into the parking lot of the liquor store.

Steve was stumbling over to pour another drink when a shooting pain penetrated his foot. He ignored it while walking by the culprits—empty bottles and take-out containers. By this point, the pounds he had lost were found again. His morning runs were kiboshed by hangovers. He had two festering fears—one was gaining his weight back. It came back all right, along with the familiar aches and pains. The following morning, Steve felt the shooting pain as he got out of bed. It was so bad he had to crawl to the washroom. Gout, also known as "The King's Disease" (painful joints), was trying to get his attention and tell him to bring back his life as he went from a fit marathoner to hobbling with a cane.

The more Steve succumbed to his feelings, the more he drank. The more he drank, the more shame and guilt he felt. The more shame and guilt, the more anger he held. Then his second biggest fear appeared—he lost the connection with his sons. The environment he had created perpetuated his fears as his angry outbursts pushed his sons away. He was turning into someone they hardly recognized. Steve's invisible trap hijacked his life. He did not have the coping skills, and they certainly didn't come with his past diet regimes. Instead, his failures added to the shame-guilt triggered cycle. For Steve to step out of his trap, he needed to let go of the shame.

AFRAID OF LETTING GO

You and I are just one thought away from an invisible trap. However, if your thoughts create a trap, they can also help you escape. Who holds the key to your toxic emotions? With all the trials and tribulations, you're often your own worst jury. Where did Steve's guilt really come from? Who decides how much and how long to carry it? Why do some seem to lock themselves up and throw away the key while others skip right past sentencing, letting go and bypassing their convictions? Meanwhile, you wrestle with yours and tighten the cuffs. Maybe you're afraid to let go too quickly because it seems heartless? Some crimes serve a determined sentence while lesser crimes can have a lifelong sentence if held in the mind. Convictions are not all bad, but remaining with them is. Either way, you get to decide, and you hold the only key, which is called perception.

Mary believed her feelings of self-loathing led to her kidney disease. Similarly, when Steve, Pamela, Mary, you, and I stay in toxic thinking, we can easily equate this to disease. Does dis-ease create disease? Thoughts become feelings, and in the physical sense, those symptoms felt by the body are trying to get your attention. Steve's angry outbursts potentially morphed into the searing symptoms of gout. If you pay attention to what the anger is telling you, you'll see anger is usually code for fear. In Steve's case, he feared losing his sons, which etched a fight-flight response into his system.

Anger can be a protective mechanism, leading us to fight to defend ourselves. With actual danger, the flee response is a necessary option. However, chronic fear isn't a good strategy or chemistry for your body to soak in. Fear skewed Steve's parenting skills, making him hold his boys with a tighter grip, which robbed them of the freedom to be with friends and created a guilt cycle for them. Everywhere Steve turned, the coals were being stirred, until the chain reaction in his body forced him to let go. Then he heard a small whisper saying, "It's time to rise again."

PICKING UP YOUR GOOD VIBRATIONS

Have you felt anger course through your veins? Feelings can be felt through and outside of you. Jack Fraser of the University of Oxford says, "Your body is made of cells containing atoms and electron charges producing a cascade of electrical signals transmitted through your body. Like nano electrical generators, sensors send signals to your brain. Every cell and organ in your body has its magnetic field emitting energy." This is precisely how some medical technologies can capture images and/or data. Emotions or "e-motions" are energy in motion, so they can be measured.

Dr. Shawna Freshwater, clinical psychologist, suggests anger, depression, and anxiety are "the most prevalent in our culture." She describes emotions as a predominant link to the mind-thought narrative about self and others. Although the measurements of your emotions may not be validated by all researchers, the following renowned doctors have documented evidence. Dr. Joe Dispenza, a famous neuroscientist and author wrote, "All energy has a frequency carrying information including your thoughts and feelings." Additionally, Dr. David Hawkins, a distinguished psychiatrist, obtained data measuring common human emotions as indicated below, which reflect similar findings in Dispenza's work.

Emotions in Hertz:

Enlightenment	700
Peace	600
Love	500
Acceptance	350
Courage	200
Anger	150
Desire	125
Fear	100
Grief	75
Guilt	30
Shame	20

Steve's emotions seemed to hover around shame (20Hz) and guilt (30Hz), the lowest on the scale of emotions. He is not alone. Experiencing these emotions is normal, but troubles come when you get stuck in them.

What Steve didn't know is anger (150Hz) measures higher than guilt. Why would anger measure higher? Perhaps it is misunderstood. Energetically, anger can lead you to one of three places: 1) Back to Guilt, 2) Stuck in Anger, or 3) Leveraging Courage (200Hz). Anger, of course, is part of the fight-flight response providing the courage to fight. In some cases, the fight is you pulling yourself up to get going again. This understanding of anger isn't about condoning it or remaining in it, but using it to rise and move on.

Can you see the emotional ties to eating when dis-ease leads to disease? Awareness can help you replace bandage food remedies that attempt to numb. It isn't about judging yourself. The hurt teen or child in you became an adult, but that doesn't automatically equip you to know how to truly heal. Nobody wants pain, and you do what you know how to do to dull it, misunderstood feelings can build walls to isolate at the same time. Not knowing how to deal with anger or grief while feeling guilt sets us up for more walls of shame.

What if just the right amount of anger came without guilt and was seen as a temporary lapse of reason? Then you might be quicker to move up to Acceptance (350Hz). According to the Gottman Institute, anger is actually a secondary emotion and code for the primary emotions like fear and hurt. Conflict itself is normal, but developing skills to handle anger and conflict is the challenge. Perhaps anger doesn't always represent what is going on underneath. Chaos can evoke change. Staying in comfort does not. In discomfort, anger, and guilt, you might be assessing your circumstances, causing yourself to grow. If you stay in comfort, you may not ask, "What would I Love (500 Hz) instead of the pain?" Upon arriving at the level of love, you cross a threshold leading to Enlightenment (700Hz).

Steve admitted that if not for the journey, he would have missed what the chaos was there to reveal. It would have remained deep down, but the discomfort caused a search for more than what the distraction of alcohol could do. Upon picking himself up and asking what he would love, good vibrations revealed even more.

> "It's better to be pulled by your dream than pushed by your pain."
>
> — Unknown

EMOTIONAL DISEASE

Your subconscious memorizes your emotions, frequency, or "set point" much like the thermostat in your home. If anger covering your hurt in fight-flight is your thermostat setting, it almost becomes defined as your personality. In a cyclical effect, using "food remedies" to "douse anger," matters are made worse. An angry person will justify their remedies as a way to relax and calm themselves. The combination of emotions and an unhealthy lifestyle can ignite more pressures, leading to high blood pressure, ulcers, acid reflux, etc. In a way, you are digesting your stress. The stress creates cortisol, increasing the risk of heart disease and weight gain. If "I defiantly deserve a drink today" (or fill in the blank) becomes a reward system, it will keep you on repeat. In fact, you might even invent stress or incite more anger to justify the next drink/reward.

Steve was looking for reasons to drink. It was his reward system since nothing else seemed to be. It was ironic, really, because compassion would have soothed his hurt, but it was disguised by anger nobody wanted to be around. However, the byproduct, gout, managed to get his attention. Many would agree a link exists between chronic disease and stress. Stress is quite subjective and everyone processes and perceives it differently; quite often it is acknowledged but still minimized. Though, suffice it to say, a holistic approach to healing, in my opinion, requires more awareness, and I believe, perhaps a little more compassion is on the horizon.

TRANSFORMING YOUR ATTITUDE ALTITUDE

What is your *attitude* set at? Do you wake up happy? Do you have patterns you're unaware of like memorizing suffering or gratitude? If you feel annoyed when someone is overly happy, who needs a rise in the "altitude on their attitude"?

Many rise in the morning on autopilot following the same routine—get up from the same side of the bed, shuffle to the washroom, brush their teeth, shower, and drive to work the same way every day. The conscious mind is hardly engaged. If your job and nighttime routine are mundane, the same "wiring is firing." If you want a different result, you have to "raise with praise" and adjust the "altitude of your attitude." Your desires for more well-being and/or to release weight require transforming your frequency since your desires are operating on the frequency of what you would *love*. It's like your radio is set on AM, but your dream is set on FM. You need to dial to a new frequency for you. You and your desire will, otherwise, stay on different frequencies. Who do you need to be or what steps do you need to take to switch to FM? Since your dream is on the frequency of "what you would love," start doing more of what you love. Being a person of gratitude will also help tune you in. In fact, gratitude and abundance are on the same frequency. As Patrick Snow, author of *Creating Your Own Destiny* says, "When you want something you've never had, you have to do something you've never done, and if you want what others have, you may have to do what they are doing."

Setting positive intentions before going to bed and upon waking can also generate gratitude. New habits and a new domino effect are underway. When you change your "attitude altitude," new neurons grow and new connections form a whole new you with a whole new view.

"Your moods are determined by your subconscious mind. The sum of your previous experience and feelings usually determines them."

— Raymond Charles Barker

FROM WORRIER TO WARRIOR

> "Worry is like a rocking chair: It gives you something to do but never gets you anywhere."
>
> — Erma Bombeck

Joan, a twenty-nine-year-old cashier, struggled with irritable bowel disease. She was quite frail, with thinning hair and pale skin. A recent bout of diverticulitis (an infection in the bowel) had exacerbated her intolerance to dairy, which topped her long list of food restrictions, and she lost twenty pounds. Overall, Joan was malnourished. She felt anger watching her family or colleagues enjoy the foods she loved but could not indulge in. Although she was on her feet all day, and needed the nourishment, she feared the repercussions of eating. She arrived home each evening starving only to see her favorite foods beseeching her from the pantry. All too often, it meant another cookie binge to temporarily slake her appetite, offering pleasure despite the pain and guilt afterward. Each time she cried, "Why do I do this to myself? I know better." Sound familiar?

Joan eventually joined a program that offered support from a dietitian, life coach, and yoga instructor. Joan was able to pinpoint the root cause of her struggle. She found she had unknowingly developed a pattern of worry that added pressure to all aspects of her life. Her mother was a worrier and had a poor relationship with food. Consequently, and subconsciously, her mother-controlled Joan's food intake through criticism and fear. When Joan was younger, she would sneak food to avoid her mother's glare. The paradox here is how control often backfires.

The program helped Joan lift the veil to realize she was perpetuating the same behaviors. Her love-hate relationship with controlled food intake caused disease and created more reasons to continue hiding and controlling her eating, just as her subconscious was programmed to. Once the problem was exposed, she made small changes. Since not eating at work was a form of hiding her intake as she did with her mother, she slowly shifted to eating tolerable foods at work, which meant she returned home nourished. She was not as hungry, so she binged less. Less binging meant less inflammation in her digestive system and more healing. She also improved her relationship with food, giving her more stamina, which soon led to a promotion at work. It was an attitude transformation from "worrier to warrior."

SHOULD OR SHOULD NOT

What happens when you tell your teenager to avoid something "bad"? Do they always listen? Did you? Your inner child, and especially your inner teenager, doesn't like restrictions and wants freedom. When Joan was restricted as a child, it backfired. Unless you learned how to fall, get back up, and conquer temptation in your teens, how can you automatically expect to know how to do it in adulthood? As an adult, you have the freedom to choose without looming parents, but that doesn't mean you learned how. You already know eating the whole cake or pizza is a bad idea—this isn't about education. It is about control and how you function under rules when you are overwhelmed.

Too many restrictions can make you feel trapped, triggered, and ready to explode into another binge. Some eat/binge fast enough to bypass the argument over "should or should not." You don't want to be talked out of your pleasures. The teenager in you would rather break a rule, experience pleasure (reward), and be grounded afterward than be forbidden. The DNA of your inner cave dweller has already made sacrifices and followed restrictions. After a taste of freedom, why would you want to be trapped again? If your guilt-diet cycle serves salads as punishment, you risk resenting healthy foods too. Relationships succeed by compromise, not rules. Give yourself permission occasionally to savor a piece of good quality chocolate while being guilt-free. Have strawberries and ice cream in a special crystal bowl by candlelight—celebrate.

The guilt's not working anyway. What have you got to lose? Get creative!

> "Creative ideas can never make their appearance through unhappy states of mind."
>
> — Raymond Charles Barker

Domino Diet Moment

Guilt/Worry Thoughts⇨Fight-Flight⇨Anger⇨Fall⇨Guilt/Worry⇨Symptoms ⇨Trap

Acceptance Thoughts⇨R&R⇨Compassion⇨Rising⇨New Levels ⇨Love ⇨Freedom

REFLECTIONS

1. What is your average attitude frequency on the Hertz spectrum?

   _____

   _____

   _____

   _____

2. Where do you still hold anger? Is it calling you to move up to what you love? What would you love?

   _____

   _____

   _____

   _____

ACTION STEP

Take a few minutes in the morning to "raise with praise" to enhance your vibration. It helps to think about or write down three things you are grateful for and proud of. Bob Proctor, motivational speaker and author, suggests saying what you are grateful for, waiting five minutes to listen for guidance in your day, and then sending love to three people you are upset with as a way to dial up your day. Don't forget to use an affirmation (see below) with your conscious mind when you wake and/or while brushing your teeth and before bed. Place sticky notes by your toothbrush and around the house as reminders.

SUMMARY

Feelings are powerful, but they are fourth in line in the Domino Formula. They are a byproduct of hormones stemming from your thoughts. Regardless, they can either prompt you to act or keep you in a trap. Emotions not only act as a catalyst for your thoughts; they also emit energy. Emotions are the language of the body and are often there to get your attention. Raising your vibrational frequency with new routines can help you dial up toward your dream. If you love your results, then you're on the right path. If not, make one small change in your routine by becoming aware of your thoughts, feelings, and patterns. Know your emotions and how they can assist or derail you. Observe without judgment, since even anger may be there to help you move forward. Most have not been taught how to fall and rise—but now you are more aware. What part of you is seeking to emerge? What would you love?

AFFIRMATION

"Every day, in every way, I'm getting better and better."

— Emile Coue

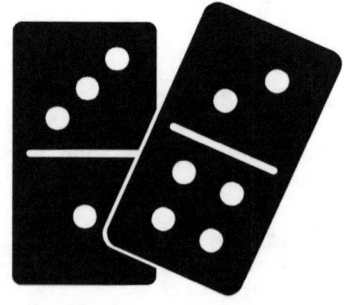

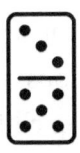

CHAPTER 8

EXPOSING YOUR FEARS

"There are only two primary emotions, fear and love."

— *A Course in Miracles*

Do you fear success? When you succeed, do you then manage to sabotage it—like managing your sugars, feeling great, and then binging on ice cream—but don't know why? Why achieve what you love and later knock it down?

Your fear of success runs far and deep. Once again, your DNA is protecting you by using fear. Today, fear (false evidence appearing real) is often a mix of *past* thoughts of unworthiness and failures and *future* thoughts anticipating pain. Past traumas drag along into adulthood, often feeding on poor coping skills that try to bury fears, hoping they fade into the sunset. However, with every sunset, there is a sunrise, and fear energy will eventually rise too. You may unknowingly eat or drink your fear as a knee-jerk reaction, but you now know you must "expose to dispose" of them.

Exposing fear through awareness is only one step, though. Think of individuals diagnosed with lung cancer who keep smoking. Awareness is not enough. With your conscious mind, however, you can kill fear with kindness. Love, after all, is on a higher frequency than fear. Since the subconscious works well with repeated thoughts, consciously using empowering affirmations can help replace and dispose old fears.

Let's expose your hidden barriers to success by using the combined wisdom of Mat Boggs, executive director of the Brave Thinking Institute, and Gay Hendricks, author of *The Big Leap*. They note that there are four hidden barriers to success.

FOUR BARRIERS TO SUCCESS

1. **Feeling Fundamentally Flawed:** Not feeling good enough, fear of judgment and/or rejection. At the root, you've wanted to fit in since birth. In fact, your DNA is programmed to fit in for survival. Being rejected from the pack meant being out in the cold, a vulnerable target. For centuries, being accepted was life or death. Now it's just fearing critics, judgment, and/or inferiority. You may even fear being too fit or losing weight because you fear it will change your relationships.

   Signs and Symptoms:
   - You fear friends won't accept you if you say no to alcohol.
   - You point out your flaws before others, thinking it will hurt less.
   - You want to start jogging, but you worry what the neighbors will think.
   - You clean your house before your hired cleaner arrives.
   - You are addicted to perfectionism and fear judgment.

- You reach a goal but fear growth and leaving your comfort zone.

Positive Repatterning: I love this quote by Theodore Roosevelt: "It is not the critic who counts…the credit belongs to the man who is actually in the arena, whose face is marred by dust and sweat and blood, who strives valiantly, who errs, who comes short again and again…and who at worst, if he fails, at least he fails while daring greatly." There are critics, but there are also risk-takers and trend-setters who pave the paths for others. No one escapes fear completely, but when you move forward with progress, instead of waiting for perfection, you might lead the pack in the end.

2. **Fear of Outshining:** You might fear outgrowing or outshining your parents, family, friends, or coworkers. You fear feeling superior while others feel inferior. You might fear appearing too selfish or greedy, which means you secretly believe in lack or a limited supply. At the root, there is also the primal fear of being rejected, leaving you thinking if you surpass others, you might be exiled while the pack maintains its alliances.

    Signs/Symptoms:
    - You play small to avoid outgrowing your relationships.
    - You avoid appearing smart so others won't feel inferior.
    - You feel uncomfortable with accolades or being the center of attention.
    - You talk more about your failures than your successes.
    - You fear having more money or things or a larger home than your friends.
    - You want to run a marathon but fear your friends will sneer.

Positive Repatterning: Keep growing. The world needs inventors and those willing to reach farther. You and I would still be using horses and plows otherwise. Risk-takers find cures and become heroes. There is no shortage of abundance. There is an unlimited supply for everyone who takes a step. Poverty doesn't help anyone advance, but riches sure can. Be a diamond in the rough; diamonds have flaws but still shine.

3. **Fear the Burden of Success:** This fear is also known as fear of burnout or having less freedom because of the commitments that accompany success. You might fear joining a gym and/or changing routines, for instance. If you reached success previously and fell, you might fear trying again.

   Signs/Symptoms:
   - Thinking you've already peaked or your good days are behind you.
   - Thinking you don't have time—code for being too scared to try again.
   - Thinking you won't be able to have fun anymore if you commit to a health program.
   - Thinking it will cost too much (gyms, equipment, eating healthy, new clothes) or fear of gaining too much bulk if you exercise.

   Positive Repatterning: Olympic athletes, billionaires, and so on all take breaks. Aim for quality over quantity with workouts and food. Do what you love, and it will naturally balance in other areas, including rest. You deserve a life you love.

4. **Fear of Abandonment:** Looking fit, being the healthy one, or looking different can mean risking abandonment by family, friends, or coworkers.

   Signs/Symptoms:

   - You join your friends on the weekend out of guilt despite your schedule.
   - You stay later than you intended because of peer pressure.
   - You eat what friends eat and drink, even though you'd rather not.
   - You gossip with friends, even if you don't agree.
   - You fear charging for your services and tell yourself it's okay, despite resentment.
   - You are a people pleaser/caregiver who puts others' needs before your own to the point of exhaustion; you forget to put your own oxygen mask on first.

   Positive Repatterning: "In a relaxed and easy manner, everything required is being accomplished in ways that feel really good to me for the highest good of all concerned," says Kirsten Welles, master coach of the Brave Thinking Institute.

You might have noticed the overlap in these barriers to success—they are intertwined in ways that are difficult to separate. For instance, you can fear the *burden of success* and *abandonment* at the same time. In any case, one may stand out more, and therefore, a certain affirmation may also stand out. Revisit these fears often and pay attention to your thoughts as they guide you.

> "A wolf need not be concerned with the opinions of sheep."
>
> — Unknown

Domino Diet Moment

Fear Thoughts ⇒ Fight-Flight ⇒ Fear Feelings ⇒ Hidden Triggers ⇒ Stay Small ⇒ Disease

Positive Thoughts ⇒ R&R ⇒ Gratitude ⇒ Trendsetter ⇒ Proud ⇒ Dreams ⇒ Health Harmony

REFLECTIONS

1. Which of the four fears of success do you see in your self-sabotaging patterns?

   _____
   _____
   _____
   _____

2. What fears are holding you back?

   _____
   _____
   _____
   _____

ACTION STEP

Write a customized affirmation to kick fear in the rear. Then take a step toward your goals. As Dale Carnegie said, "If you want to conquer fear, do not sit home and think about it. Go out and get busy." Taking a step is a way of repatterning too.

SUMMARY

Fear tries to hold you back and govern your success in many ways. Fear of judgment, opinions, failure, and hurt may seem obvious, but at the root are hidden fears and self-sabotage learned as far back as your childhood and running as deeply as your very DNA. Don't be afraid to expose what is trying to hide in the dark. Becoming aware is a step and conscious affirmations can shine a light on what you love.

> "You cannot chase away the dark, but you can turn on a light."
>
> — Mary Morrissey

AFFIRMATION

Fear is a liar; love is my desire.

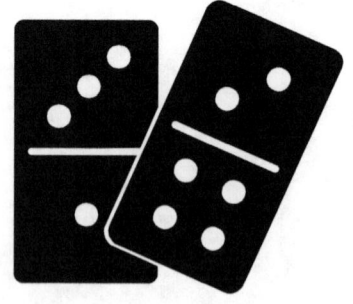

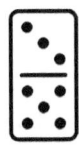

CHAPTER 9

LOVE HERTZ

"There are only two primary emotions, fear and love."

— *A Course in Miracles*

I am circling back to the same quote as the previous chapter to talk about the second primary emotion—love. Despite love (500Hz) having a higher frequency than fear (100Hz) based on the spectrum of emotions in Chapter 7, sometimes it appears fear has more power because it often holds you back from what you love. Going a little deeper, you might discover the power behind love that is so feared.

Have you been hurt? Maybe suffered a breakup, rejection, or abandonment? As the band Nazareth said best, "Love Hurts."

Songs have a way of speaking in a language of their own. They can instantly send you traveling nostalgically through your teens, breakups, weddings, tears, and laughter. Songs can stir emotions, and they can also heal them. Sounds, rhythm, and words can all strike a chord. In fact, music therapists study-specific vibrations and sounds to determine which ones provide a healing frequency or the opposite. Think of times when a song has gotten on your nerves or someone sang off-key compared to a song that soothes you. Songs have a way of speaking straight to the heart, bypassing the left brain's logical thinking, cutting through even in the angriest of moods.

If you place two pianos together and hit middle C on one piano, the string for middle C on the second piano will also vibrate. The Law of Vibration states that everything that moves has a vibration. Everything living has a vibration. Your body transmits and receives vibrations from your mind, your words, and the words of others, according to the Law of Vibration. The vibration moves in you and through you. The old saying, "Sticks and stones may break my bones, but names will never hurt me" isn't completely true; words and tones can indeed hurt you—but they can also soothe you.

Dr. Masaru Emoto, a Japanese scientist, revolutionized the concept of thoughts and emotions in the physical realm. He studied the molecular structure of water when exposed to specific words. In controlled studies, he used water samples in which the lab assistants spoke kind or unkind words for a specified period. Under a microscope, he noticed beautiful flower and snowflake-like crystal formations on the samples exposed to words of love, joy, and peace. However, angry, hateful, and ugly words produced darker, oddly formed crystals. These results appear to indicate that water reflects the vibrations of words.

What is the significance?

Your body is 70 percent water. The vibrations of your words and feelings transmit through your body. Your corpus callosum, between your right and left brain hemispheres, contains fluid that moves through your body, including your nervous system and your cells. This means your words may carry weight and a frequency that can either lead to healthy harmony or disease.

> "All the water in the world cannot drown
> you unless it gets inside you."
>
> — Eleanor Roosevelt

LOVE LAYERS

I was four years old and sitting camouflaged in the tall grass, mesmerized by the kids in the park. I watched a young couple in their teens chasing each other around as they giggled and playfully flirted. They looked to be in love. I was four; how would I know? Maybe there is a recognizable synchronic harmony connecting love to each of us on a deeper level. Nevertheless, I blissfully watched their enchanting antics and made an internal vow to have that one day too. I didn't realize love had so many layers, though, nor did I realize my desire for love would hurt me the most.

> "The pain started so many years ago, but I'd lived with it for so long at that point that I'd accepted it as an inevitable part of me."
>
> — Ashley D. Wallis

My internal vow to find love made me vulnerable. I didn't know what love really looked like, but I sure craved it. I was like the ugly duckling searching for its mother, asking the cow, the pig, the fish, "Are you my mother?" I, instead, was asking, "Are you my love?"

An older boy named William lured me into the bushes with a candy necklace. He stood at the bush-line of the park where I watched the lovers from afar. It was off-limits, though; my mother forbade me to go to the park. I thought possessing the dangling necklace would be worth disobeying my mother. He was sixteen and cunning. He introduced me to a kind of love that wasn't love at all. Rather, I was cheated and robbed of what love was supposed to feel like. Embarrassed and ashamed, I lay there shaking as he fled the scene with the necklace still in his hands.

No necklace and no love. Instead, I felt stupid and betrayed. My four-year-old mind told me *I did something wrong*, and so I ran straight to my room. I hid, fearing my mother's wrath—I had disobeyed her by being in the woods, after all.

Mom had a way of knowing when things weren't right, so she managed to extract my confession. Although my parents approached William's, it was the '70s and these crimes were often kept silent. The boy denied everything, and his parents went along with his lies. I buried my violated, unvalidated feelings and ended my mission to find love.

My skeleton stayed in the closet for two years until eighteen-year-old William noticed his prey playing alone. By this point, being socially awkward, I often played alone. When William invited me to play cards in his trailer in the backyard, I somehow forgot the first episode and I went with him to play the card game Crazy 8s—that was crazy all right.

Thankfully, William's brother barged in as I lay there shaking. While his brother looked bewildered, I instinctively knew it was my opportunity to bolt!

I was ashamed again. I thought, *It's all my fault*. I felt there must be something wrong with me. I added another skeleton to the closet and shut the door. My closet had termites, though, gnawing away and creating holes. From the outside, I looked stable; on the inside, I was falling apart.

What would life be like if you could just be you instead of the you behind the walls and protective disguises? Would you be afraid of love if it were not for the hurt and betrayals? Deep down, I wanted love without the fear of it, and so I kept it at arm's length.

My social awkwardness continued. At thirteen, I was rather shy while still searching for love of some kind. When I walked by the popular girls and they asked me to join, I couldn't move fast enough. I so badly craved acceptance—no way was I going to botch this. When they lit a cigarette and passed it around like some sort of initiation ritual, I knew I would have to partake to be a part of the group. I put on a disguise of enthusiasm, and while I coughed and sputtered, all I could think was, *Please don't reject me.* All it took was one puff or *drag*, as they called it, and just like that, I was accepted into the group.

ADDICTED TO LOVE

Smoking was still cool in the '80s. During school breaks, the popular kids would gather in the courtyard to smoke while the nerds gathered in the library. Were the smokers really addicted to smoking or addicted to being accepted? It was acceptance for me. Soon, the parties started, and added drinking rituals. Was it alcohol addiction, or was it for acceptance too?

I didn't enjoy alcohol, but my shy, awkward side made me follow the crowd. When I drank, I loosened up and became the fun dancing queen. Not only was I accepted, but I was also fun, and it led me to my first love.

I fell for a badass! He was a good-looking, athletic player. When he took a liking to me, I was so flattered. Because I was thirteen and had a tainted view of love, when he said, "Jump," I said, "How high?" I called it love. When he cheated with my best friend, he said, "If you really love me, you'll take me back," and so I did. When I did, I pretty much wore a sign that said, "I'll do anything for love." Anything was better than being alone, right? Like a dangling carrot, he held the golden prize of *love* out in front of me. It gave him power and control. His ego puffed up, and he cheated again. That day, the whole group piled into a car and drove off, telling me there was no room. I was rejected by the group and cried all the way home. I ended up soothing my heart with food.

This is my first memory of my using food for love. How about you?

DISCOVERING YOUR TRUE CRAVINGS

I went from a fool for love to building walls to protect me from love. Unfortunately, I didn't know it at the time. My first husband lived with my pain hidden by walls, and I lived with his. His parents divorced while we were together, leaving us both floundering to learn about love. We stayed together for love and for our daughter, friends, and family, but I developed a new love addiction called *a career*. Staying busy distracted me from seeing what was hiding. Loving me was like loving a prickly rose bush—you had to go through thorns to get to me.

By now, you may have noticed a theme. Pamela, Steve, and I, and maybe you, are afraid of loneliness, rejection, hurt, and love. Many compensate and cope by building walls to keep true love out, but they allow distractions and numbing agents in as subconscious tactics to avoid being hurt again. However, there is always an escape hatch, no matter how thick your walls. Unlived passion, desires, and love are all forms of energy that search to escape, and in doing so, the energy symptomizes as a last-ditch effort to get your attention so you will allow it out. Maybe this is another reason heart disease is the number-one cause of death.

Thoughts of being left out can be replaced with a bag of chips within a split second. Habits do not come with a sign saying, "Welcome to *Emotional Eating*." Instead, they weave into the tapestry of your mind, and like they did for Pamela, they escalate until one day the emotional eater who once received pleasure numbing the pain can no longer numb it. Drama cycles within addictions work to justify your love for the distraction and cover what you're really craving. If left to its own devices, the addiction becomes your story.

THAT'S YOUR STORY—ARE YOU STICKING TO IT?

"People come into your life for a reason, a season, or a lifetime."

— Unknown

Are you addicted to your story? Is it your *true* story? Do you wish your story to be here for a season, a reason, or a lifetime?

Phyllis was a single mom with amazing twin daughters. As a devoted mother, she worked long hours, sacrificing her time to provide for her family. She had little time for a social life, being "far too busy." Coworkers invited her out, but she always said, "I'm a single mom. I don't have time. My kids need me." When her girls grew more independent, she still told the same story and would even toss it into a conversation with people she had just met. It was as if she needed to remind herself or she might forget. One day, her coworkers invited her to join them after work, confessing they had someone they wanted her to meet. As Phyllis started her usual rationalization—single mother, girls need me—in her usual negative string of words, it triggered a panic attack.

Phyllis' betrayal by her husband, who had left when the twins were born, was devastating. She adored him and what they had built together. The rejection, hurt, and fear were internalized and she had vowed never to love again. She unknowingly created a story to avoid a social life and the risk of falling in love again. Her addiction to work and becoming a hovering parent would have continued if it were not for finding a new love story.

Phyllis' aunt advised her to hire a life coach to help her focus on how to raise her daughters successfully alone and still have a life of her own. Soon, the negative imprints etched in her mind faded. Phyllis gained a whole new self-image and found love again.

Your story is filled with repeating words. Does it sound like a country song in which your spouse left you (and took the dog), or is it a song about new love? You get to decide if your story is told for a reason, a season, or a lifetime. Know this, though, as Maxwell Maltz said in *The Magic Power of Self-Image Psychology*, "You cannot outperform your own self-image."

It is true—hurt people do hurtful things, and rose-colored glasses can turn to *fifty shades of grey*. If the hurt wasn't there for me, though, I would still be with my first love and may never have found the next layer of love. With awareness, you can begin to override your subconscious and keep it from holding you back from what you would genuinely love—rather than the pretend love you get in a glass of bourbon. You can develop new ways to repattern. You have baggage; we all do. What if it is all for a prodigal son/daughter story called *Return to You*.

Remember, the subconscious doesn't know if your story is happening now, in the past, or in your imagination. You can begin to create a new movie or story with a whole new reel any time you want. Recite positive affirmations, hug the hurt—you didn't know any better; how could you? Sometimes, you need to learn the contrasts of love to know what your true love really looks like. Addictions or illnesses can teach you about disharmony. If nothing else, your discontent can begin to assess what you would love instead.

REFLECTIONS

1. What addictions do you have stemming from past trauma? List possible patterns through different periods:

    Ages 1-20 _____

    _____

    Ages 20-30 _____

    _____

    Ages 30-40 _____

    _____

    Ages 40-50 _____

    _____

Ages 50-60 _____

_____

Did your remedies serve you or hinder you?

2. Are you an emotional eater? A mindless eater? Both? What story are you broadcasting and which story would you like to be your life story?

_____
_____
_____
_____

3. Are you afraid of love? What are you being distracted from?

_____
_____
_____
_____

ACTION STEP

Rich Boggs of the Brave Thinking Institute suggests replacing your words with empowering statements as follows.

Common Negative Statements	Positive Replacements
• I have to lose weight.	• I get to choose my weight.
• I need to lose weight.	• I get to release weight.
• My doctor told me I can't have….	• I eat nourishing, whole foods.
• Healthy food costs too much.	• I invest in my health
• I have to exercise.	• I *get to* create vital dynamic health when active.
• I look at food and gain weight.	• I select foods I love that feel good to me.
• I have a bad relationship with food.	• Food nourishes me on a cellular level.
• I am a stress eater.	• I eat to nourish and fuel my day.

DOMINO DIET MOMENT

Hurt Thought⇒Breath⇒Fight-Flight⇒Fear⇒Numbing⇒Habit⇒ Behavior⇒Hurt Story

Love Thought⇒Breath⇒R&R⇒In Love⇒Affirmation⇒Habit ⇒Behavior⇒Love Story

SUMMARY

Fear and love are your two underlying emotions. It would appear once again that fear of success is in disguise—only this time it is disguised as a fear of love. The saying "Hurt people do hurtful things" is true but not limited to hurting others. Often, it refers to hurting yourself. Once upon a time, being vulnerable and chasing the dangling carrot called love may have been met with betrayal or abandonment. Unskilled handling may turn hurt into the primary emotion: fear. The fear of loving again can build walls that allow false love remedies in—just enough to keep you distracted from what you truly love. Living in the fear of love becomes a comfort zone, which the subconscious cunningly convinces you to stay in. It's like convincing yourself that lower numbers when you weigh yourself on the scale will bring happiness, but since they are often distractors from what you really want or rarely change quickly enough, you are left disappointed. Fear of love just triggers another drama cycle that justifies hiding out and indulging in numbing, counterproductive remedies that leave you exhausted, to the point you stop searching for what you truly hunger for. Soon addictions and drama become words uttered in a string that becomes your story.

The path to optimal health requires uncovering your fears and addictions by taking up residency in your own mind. Knowing you are self-sabotaging and no longer blaming friends for guilting you into dessert can be liberating. Your story reflects your self-image, and since you cannot outperform your self-image, it begins with a search for love. Fear had its turn; it's not working. Instead, stay curious about your desires and you will hear a whisper of hope. Love has more power than fear, despite your vacillation between them. Look deep and you might see loneliness is what you really fear. The fear of success often points to not wanting to be alone.

Create a new story. Attune to what is guiding you toward harmony. Mind your words and stay in the question, "What would I love?" while knowing your purpose lies there.

What story would you like to carry for a lifetime? Your past story was a chapter, not your whole book. It is your turn to turn yourself toward love.

AFFIRMATION

I choose my thoughts, my words, my story, my destiny, and what I love!

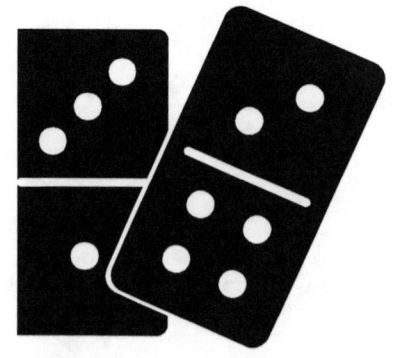

SECTION 5

BETWEEN THE FOURTH AND FIFTH DOMINO— TRANSFORMING YOU

The Domino Diet Formula

Thoughts⇨Breath⇨Hormones⇨**Feelings**[⇦⇨]**Actions**⇨Results⇨Freedom

---

"A caterpillar can fly but not as a caterpillar."

— Mary Morrissey

You have come to the section in the Domino Diet Formula that represents a space between, where ideas and dreams are at risk of being trapped. It is where feelings dictate actions, be it toward the results you desire or otherwise. Truthfully, there is no such thing as a complete pause. You create results one way or the other by merely continuing to think and breathe. Just like when you come to a fork in the road, you decide which way to go in your transformation.

According to most dictionaries, the word *transformation* includes the meaning "a metamorphosis during a life cycle of an animal" or *Meta*-Self, *Morph*-Change, *Osis*-Action. When I hear the word metamorphosis, I think of a caterpillar changing into a butterfly. Yet, truly, the metamorphosis itself is neither the caterpillar nor the butterfly. It is called a chrysalis. The chrysalis is the form between caterpillar and butterfly. One might think it is like hibernation or a pause—with the butterfly awaiting the freedom to fly—but there is more going on. The transformation is a release of old ways and the anticipation of new ones.

A young person walking in a wooded area noticed a cocoon with a butterfly trying to break free. It struggled for a while, then stopped. Saddened, the young person decided to speed up the process by relieving some of the burden and cutting the cocoon open. Instantly, the butterfly was free to fly, but it fell to the ground instead. What appeared to be a struggle cracking open the cocoon was really the wings pressing against the cocoon to release a liquid that fuses with the wings, providing the butterfly with the strength to fly.

Struggle is part of life. Are you still in your cocoon? Are you in a metamorphosis or ready to transform? Do you have a loved one who is struggling and you just want to take their burden from them so they can be free? Would that rob them of their potential transformation? You can get them support from someone who will understand without interfering while you strengthen your wings during your transformation. Many diet programs do the opposite—their quick approaches leave your wings weakened and unprepared for struggle. A healthy diet as a way of life takes more time, but with support, you'll fly to freedom in the end.

The following chapters are somewhat different than previous chapters. You will be taking steps within your transformation. You will push off boundaries and strengthen your wings. This is the place between staying stuck with your feelings and using them to act and fly from your "comfort cocoon." If you remain stuck, procrastination, excuses, fear of change, or fear of letting go all reside there. If you say, "I'm confused about where to start," it is another form of distraction keeping you stuck. Confusion is the cousin of delay. This is also where "I'm not good enough," "I already tried that," "I don't have time," or "I'm too old" lies and delays your transformation. You can move forward, though. Wing it. Break free. You are stronger than you think.

> "Our borders and our obstacles can only do two things: 1) stop us in our tracks, or 2) force us to get creative. It's not about breaking down borders, it's about pushing off of them. True disability is only in our mind."
>
> — Amy Purdy

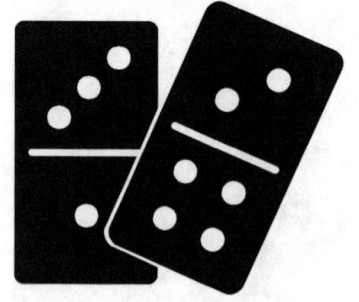

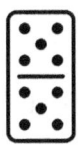

CHAPTER 10
FINDING YOUR FREEDOM

"In the truest sense, freedom cannot be bestowed; it must be achieved."

— Franklin D. Roosevelt

It didn't seem outlandish at fifteen to own my first car, but it was out of my reach at thirteen when the desire for freedom started to arise. I wanted to be at the mall with friends or hanging at a house listening to tunes, but it meant asking for a ride. I saved $400 by making three dollars an hour. My parents matched that. On my sixteenth birthday, I drove my $800, 1976 Pinto, leaving my cocoon, and flew to freedom! Do you remember your first day of freedom?

I imagined driving, feeling the steering wheel, hearing the music blaring, the wind coming in the open windows, and no parents! Throughout life, you have been consciously and subconsciously sowing and reaping results. Below are steps many of the authors quoted in this book advise as tools to create more consistently positive outcomes:

1. Decide on what you want and define it clearly and specifically, visualizing it with mental pictures.
2. Visualize the results you want as though they have already come to pass using your five senses.
3. Set a deadline and revisit your vision morning and night.
4. Take steps with what you have, from where you are now.
5. Be open to results outside your plan—they may be something even better still.

A study published in the *Journal of Behavioral Science* on Episodic Future Thinking suggests using your imagination to visualize your dream with as many pictures as possible to get maximum buy-in from your brain. Picture your ideal relationship, health, or any dream as if you are living it now. Remember, your subconscious doesn't know the difference when your conscious mind repeats imagined results. The more specific the vision, the more senses you use, the more emotions you engage, and the more episodes of visioning you include, the better. When you imagined your first vehicle, did you imagine driving with the windows down, etc.? Did you imagine it using all five senses?

What would you love? Picture your dream home or optimal fitness as if you already have it. A GPS, when driving, doesn't say, "No, sorry; you can't drive to New York." It simply uploads the data. Your subconscious does the same. It will require specificity, though, as in, "Where in New York City?" Similarly, saying, "I want a lot of money," will not work. You need more specifics since you can't cash a check for "a lot of money." Declaring I want vital, dynamic health instead of I want to lose weight is a more empowering way of reaching your goal. You do not need to know how it will all happen just as you don't always know every mile or turn of the road when planning to drive to a destination. You will be guided along the way much like your GPS reveals more as you go, and as you take steps, your subconscious mind opts-in, knowing you mean business and will help take you to your dream too.

> "Freedom is not worth having if it does not include
> the freedom to make mistakes."
>
> — Mahatma Gandhi

DRIVING OUT OF BALANCE

When Mom and Dad helped with my sky-blue '76 Pinto purchase, the deal was Dad was granted permission to deliver his sermon on "mechanical safety" before I left the nest to freedom. Off we drove as Dad instructed me on adjusting mirrors, checking the oil, watching for warning lights, and listening for sounds. The only sound I wanted to hear was the boom of my stereo. Overly excited, I managed to tune out most of his advice. Like a stereotypical teen, I knew it all anyway. He said something about, "Don't ignore warning signs because it will cost more in the end."

Finally, while on my own at a later date, I was driving somewhere in a rush when I thought I heard a clunk, but the music was blaring, so I ignored it and carried on. Then the clank and clunk tried to get my attention, but I was almost where I was going and pressed on. Just before I reached my destination, I heard the fizz, splat that left me stranded. I was too distracted and had missed or ignored the warning signs, so I ended up driving out of balance. Dad was right—ignoring warnings can cost more in the end. Are you out of balance?

Bill enjoyed his truck-driving career. His scenic territory took him home every night to be with his family. New management, however, made changes, creating longer hours and less time at home. It started slowly, but Bill developed a severe rash that covered his entire body. It made for painful showers and sleep. Soon, he couldn't drive long periods either. Worse, though, was that his deflating self-esteem was starting to affect his relationship.

Bill tried eliminating foods. His diet became so restricted that the quality of his life declined—his symptoms remained, and depression set in. His work schedule made it more difficult to eat healthy, and after spending thousands on medications, ointments, and appointments, he came to a dead end. Finally, one day as he arrived at work, he noticed a suffocating feeling. He thought, *Am I allergic to work?* He admitted he felt like he was checking his soul at the door at work and picking it up on the way home. Bill's disease was trying to get his attention, but he ignored the first warning light, which cost him more in the end. His inner GPS tried to get him to recalculate, but he wasn't listening.

Aches and pains, digestive issues, tightness in the chest, allergic reactions—pay attention to your warning signs. Are you going the wrong way? What will it cost you in the end? Let's do an assessment to see how to "balance you to freedom."

> "Let yourself be silently drawn by the strange pull or what you really love. It will not lead you astray."
>
> — Rumi

ASSESSING YOUR BALANCE

The Brave Thinking Institute and the special *Time Magazine* edition, *The Science of Success*, suggest your happiness and whole well-being is rooted in four areas: love, health, career, and time/money freedom. Much like four wheels on your vehicle, neither one is more important than the other, and they are all interconnected. If one wheel is overinflated or underinflated, your vehicle is out of balance. If you have money but no time or someone to share it with, are you balanced? If you focus only on your career, do you risk your health and relationships?

When you take your car for a mechanical inspection, does the mechanic just look under the hood? Of course not, because they know a complete inspection is the only way to obtain a full diagnosis. While Bill had lab work done to "check the oil," a full inspection was missing. Finally, with the help of a dietitian and life coach, Bill completed a full assessment by rating the four areas mentioned above. On a scale of one to five, with one being extremely unhappy and five being extremely happy, his assessment went something like this....

Assessment/Rating:

Health:	3
Career:	1
Relationships:	4
Time/Money:	3

Although at first it appeared his rash was what led to the assessment in the first place, his health was rated higher than he would have originally thought. In his mind since a rash wasn't as severe as cancer, he rated his health accordingly. Surprisingly, though, his career knocked things out of balance. It turns out his rash coincided with changes at work and his fears of being away from home, fears that resulted from his father being away from home, which had affected their relationship and his father's health. He realized he was reliving his childhood, worrying about being a father who wasn't there during his son's formative years.

Bill had a dream deep down that had been trying to get his attention all along, but he pressed on with responsibilities, the paycheck, and health benefits. Still, it was costing him to the point of exhaustion and burnout.

DEFINING BURNOUT

Are you afraid to dream and put yourself out there? Do you feel too old to start over or fear another burnout?

One time, I was working for a prestigious organization on a six-year contract. The job involved flying to meetings, which I enjoyed, but it also meant often being away from my daughter. With only three months left to go on the contract's term, everything went sideways. The international conference in South Africa was supposed to be a reward at the end of my term. But the reward would also highlight my burnout and provide a U-turn for me.

When I woke up in my hotel room, intending to get ready for my long-awaited conference, I sat up and could hardly move. It felt like I was sinking through the mattress while my head was being sucked through a tunnel. All I could think was, *You've looked forward to this for years. What the heck is wrong?* I scanned my mind for all the possible reasons—jet lag, the wine, my three-week-old marriage separation on its way to divorce, or recovery from a recent marathon. It was a culmination of everything, I'm sure, but I could not see that at the time.

I managed to force myself to walk toward the conference, but a gravitational pull dragged me in the opposite direction. I wandered in a daze, drifting through the maze of markets in Cape Town. While listlessly sauntering through the aisles of artifacts and souvenirs, I overheard someone say, "This DVD saved me. I need two more please! This DVD is amazing." In my desperation, I bought one, somehow snapped out of my lethargy, and dashed to my room.

I plopped the DVD into my computer. Light surged through me as images of ancient books flashed on the screen. The narrator, Rhonda Byrne, announced the title with a mystic whisper—*The Secret*. I was fixated and, at the same time, a choir sang outside my window in a park across the way. Like a perfect duet, *The Secret* and the outside music reached a blissful place inside of me and elevated me to a whole new level. I had no idea the light in me was dimming in the first place.

Most people recognize cold or flu symptoms, but not the warning signs of burnout. The pure exhaustion, the brain fog, the lost desire for things you normally love, insomnia, anxiety, depression, resentment, etc. The challenge is burnout can disguise itself as your retreat to a comfy cocoon. For me, it was an ironclad cocoon suffocating my true dream. I honestly believed my path, despite the sacrifices, would help me build my peak career as a dietitian. The plan was going smoothly until that day.

The disappointment of the fall, though, held me captive for some time until I realized it would require a fall of that magnitude to get my attention. If I had attended the conference that day in mild discomfort, my light may have dimmed even further, or worse, it may have symptomized. I would have pressed on, ignoring my inner GPS and clunking sounds.

The DVD was the beginning of my U-turn. It was my first true embracing of the concept of the Law of Attraction. Looking back, it is quite possible it also provided a hope of creating a whole new world since mine was unravelling.

Please note, if you are suffering from burnout, handle it with care. Set small goals since big ones may have burnt you out in the first place. Do one self-care act a day as an act of kindness for yourself. Seek support and/or more information on my website (www.TheDominoDiet.com).

MAKING A "YOU" TURN

> "Time is what we want most but what we use worst."
>
> — William Penn

Did raising kids or tending to elderly parents put *you* on hold? Are you saying you don't have time, which is code for something else? No one knows when they will hit the pillow for the last time. Do you have things left undone or a legacy to leave behind? Is it time to make a *you-*turn?

In a study, 100 elderly patients in palliative care were asked what they regretted most. More than 90 percent said they regretted the things they did not do more than things they did. Why would so many leave so much undone? Once again, it comes down to *fear*. Were you stopped by the fear of failure, judgment, being too old, too young, under-resourced (time/money), and fear of commitment? All fears wrapped in the past where dreams never fly and stay to die! John Boggs, CEO of the Brave Thinking Institute, suggests three powerful questions to help remove fear roadblocks.

1. Is there anyone you need to resolve matters with?
2. Did you experience all you intended and live a full life?
3. Are you proud of who you are?

Did you know that if you live to be eighty, you will have spent more than 700,000 hours on this planet? More spend time thinking about money than the most precious currency—*time*. Time is something that once spent, you do not get back. Therefore, where you invest your time matters. Making a *you*-turn and assessing your time can be powerful. For instance, if you are fifty years old and live to be eighty, you have about 262,000 hours left to create your legacy. You still have time. Saying, "I don't have time" isn't completely true. You might even feel motivated to find ways to live even longer.

When Bill assessed the four main areas of his life and discovered his dream, he realized, at fifty, he still had time. All along, Bill wanted his own trucking company that he and his son could own and operate. It would be a legacy to leave behind, allowing him to have what he missed with his father. His time assessment also dialed up his dream to improve his health for the journey and look for ways to live even longer. He became like an auctioneer, "Who will give me thirty, thirty-five, forty more years?" How can you improve and maybe extend your time to do what you love? First, identify what keeps you stuck.

NEED A TOW?

Maybe your health dreams have changed over the years and your desire for a bikini/speedo body doesn't incentivize you the same anymore. When *vanity* dials down from a boil to a simmer, leaving your *vitality* to pick up the slack, that is when the rubber meets the road. Vitality may not have the same luster if you've lost hope or feel your best days are behind you. Who could blame you? The focus on vanity has been distracting the majority of people from following their true dreams for years. There is a way, though. If you latch on to your true dream, your desire will dial up again and tow along the rest of you.

Bill stayed at his job long enough to save for a used truck and then started his company. His focus became the company and the desire for vitality. Bill inflated his career, and it just so happened his health improved too. Having his own schedule and territory allowed him to be home and follow a healthier schedule while dialing down fear and stress. Carrying nourishing foods with him replaced truck stop foods, and more time at home allowed him and his wife to walk and do yoga. As stress cleared, his rash did too.

If you are attempting to achieve optimal health but appear blocked in getting there, chances are the dream isn't big enough or you need something bigger to latch onto. I confess my bias is on health as the tire to inflate first. Even if you have all the money in the world, without your health, where will you spend it? Without health, can you still enjoy your time or relationships?

When I assessed my time, career, health, and relationships, I realized it was time for me to realign too. The DVD took me in a circuitous route that eventually helped me latch onto a dream that emerged, which was bigger than what I thought I was doing. I had a legacy to leave behind even though I hadn't known it. Take a step; your destination is ahead.

> "A journey of a thousand miles begins with one step."
>
> — Lao Tzu

DOMINO DIET MOMENT

Un-Balanced Thoughts⇒Fight-Flight⇒Anxious Feelings⇒Fear Blocks⇒Symptoms

Balanced Thoughts⇒R&R⇒Calm Feelings⇒Actions Steps⇒Dream Results

REFLECTIONS

1. Have you been putting yourself on hold? Does your health goal need a tow? What possible sounds/knocks are trying to get your attention?

   _____
   _____
   _____
   _____

2. Have you faced burnout? Were there signs? List the ways burnout helped you and the ways it might still be holding you back.

   _____
   _____
   _____
   _____

ACTION STEP

Take a moment to assess the four areas of your life listed below using a scale of one to five, with one being extremely unhappy; two, unhappy; three, somewhat happy; four, happy; five, extremely happy.

Health:
Relationships:
Time/Money:
Career:

Side note: Time/Money is often in the same category to represent freedom. For more questions and to help customize your assessment, refer to my website (www.TheDominoDiet.com) for support.

SUMMARY

Do you have a dream and/or a legacy to leave behind? Are you still in the midst of your metamorphosis? Don't let confusion, the cousin of delay, stand in the way of taking steps. Assess the four deep-rooted areas of fulfilled happiness in your life—health, relationships, career, and time/money freedom—and you might discover a dream to latch onto. You can always adjust your course as you go, but a journey of 1,000 miles still begins with one step, even if you have to stop and rest now and then. Time is too precious to waste. It is a currency you will not get back. Invest wisely, leaving no regrets while you transform your way to freedom, growing new wings to fly.

> "Just when the caterpillar thought the world was over, it became a butterfly."
>
> — Unknown

Tip: Write a description of what your dream life looks like as though it is already happening. Take some time and put in as much detail as possible. It might be a few pages. Then create a travel-size version on one page to look at and read out loud daily.

AFFIRMATION

I am vibrant in dynamic health; I have all the energy required to serve my dreams!

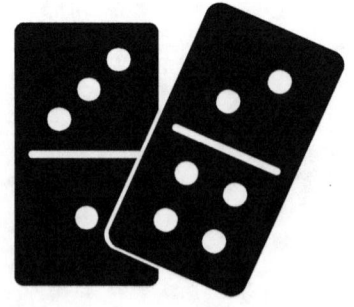

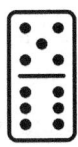

CHAPTER 11

SURVIVING THE SCHOOL OF HARD KNOCKS

"The school of hard knocks is an accelerated curriculum."

— Menander

I had it backward. You know the saying, "I come from the school of hard knocks." I believed it had to be true for me, but I also believed it was due to being flawed somehow. Yet, who hasn't had a few knocks? If you have success, you've had a few falls; it's as though it is a prerequisite to success. Place your attention on what matters, as in the rise from a fall. Ask yourself if you can rise without a fall. What are you rising from if not a fall?

I love this quote by Denis Waitley, author of *The Psychology of Winning*:

> Failure should be our teacher, not our undertaker. Failure is a delay, not defeat. Failure is a temporary detour, not a dead end. Failure is something we can avoid only by saying nothing, doing nothing, and being nothing.

In my humble opinion, the real failure is not in trying or falling—it is staying in the failure. Movies often use the comeback, the hero's journey, and/or the rising phoenix story since most cheer for the person trying in the face of adversity over the person with victory handed to them. In fact, is there a victory without starting out with a failure? Thomas Edison, in his 10,000 attempts to bring light with the incandescent bulb, said, "I have not failed. I've just found 10,000 ways that won't work." Often, respect is given to those who take feedback and rise up to try again. However, do you give yourself the same grace as a hero in surviving your knocks?

BOXING WITH DESTINY

> "Successful people fail on their way to success."
>
> — Bob Proctor

Two opponents, Dream Achiever and Fearful Paradigm, have been boxing for decades. Typically, Dream comes in strong between the first and third rounds, but Fearful ends up winning in the end. The last match was no different, leaving Dream contemplating throwing in the towel for good. But Dream's trainer recommended a coach. Although Dream's trainer coached him for decades, Dream's dream needed added support. Dream's new coach taught new ways and new moves. Studying his opponent also helped Fearful develop more confidence.

The day arrived for the boxers to come face to face again. Round one started, and Dream Achiever came in with a new left hook, giving Fearful Paradigm a wake-up call. The agitated Fearful came back swinging harder, but Dream took the hit and managed to bounce back swinging.

After round three, Dream was still in the game—getting further than ever before. Now, with more confidence, Dream pulled out a new move, jabbing into Fearful's blind spot. Boom! Fearful went down in the fifth round!

If you have not guessed, these two boxers are you. You are a dream achiever but may have fearful paradigms, but with support and by learning new tools, you can also conquer your fears. It is common to rise in passion and work hard, but just when it gets a little harder, to let fear and self-sabotage rise, keeping you playing small. Often, just when you are close to conquering paradigms, things become more agitated. The good news is you have a fighting chance—if you learn to spot the paradigm's blind spots.

> "Obstacles don't have to stop you. If you run into a wall, don't turn around and give up. Figure out how to climb it, go around it, or work around it."
>
> — Michael Jordan

PARADIGMS 101

When you learn the language of your dream achiever and your fear paradigm, you can decide to repattern them. Paradigms are patterns of thinking, be they positive or negative.

Fear Paradigm Language:

I will start my workouts once all the junk food is gone. It's all or nothing.

I will start Monday or after Christmas or....
I don't have time.
I don't like cooking.
It's too hot, too cold, too rainy....
I'm not a morning person.
I'm too tired after work.
I'm too busy with kids.
I'm on my feet all day.
My body doesn't like exercise.
My family won't eat healthy, and I refuse to cook two meals.
Note: The underlying root of these paradigms is fear of change.

New Dream Achiever Language

I enjoy foods I love. My motto is quality over quantity.
Everyone has the same twenty-four hours in a day. I spend time wisely and actively.
I enjoy creative ways of cooking easy, healthy meals.
I enjoy a variety of activities indoors and outdoors.
I find ways to be active through the day.
I feel energized and uplifted when I'm active.

> "Change is the essence of life. Be willing to surrender what you are for what you could become."
>
> — Unknown

How do you overcome adversity? Are you still punishing yourself or others? Whether it's a failed marriage, illness, or bankruptcy, no one escapes unscathed. Deciding to change is hardly an overnight process, but your history is not your destiny. Suffice it to say, staying in the doom and gloom headspace puts you at risk for emotional eating.

Learning a new language can help you overcome victimhood and/or blaming others. Once you learn new, positive paradigms, you are on your way to understanding your contribution to the problem, which also means you are a contributor to the solution. When you take ownership of your results, something unexpected begins to happen—you feel less captive to fear and an epiphany unfolds as you realize your mistakes are there for a reason, and they are calling you to grow and change.

SCHOOLING ON CHANGE

> "Growth is painful, change is painful, but nothing is as painful as staying stuck somewhere you don't belong."
>
> — Unknown

In the late 1970s, James Prochaska and Carlo DiClemente suggested in the transtheoretical model (TTM) that there are five phases in change as described below, using exercise as an example.

Precontemplation ⇒ Contemplation ⇒ Preparation ⇒ Action ⇒ Maintenance

Precontemplation: This phase is also known as denial. There is no intention to change, for example, "My body doesn't like exercise or gyms." This is where pressure tactics don't work. In fact, they can cause more denial and resentment. You'll know if you feel resentment if you see someone jogging or ordering a salad and roll your eyes. You might notice yourself looking for reasons not to exercise. Fear of change, sacrifice, losing favorite foods, or facing an illness often linger here. This phase requires extra compassion. Someone else's success story of overcoming a painful journey or watching documentaries with similar stories can often start an awakening.

Contemplation: You might hear a success story of someone who began exercising. You see their results and contemplate starting someday. This is good news, but approach with caution. Diet propaganda can be attractive in this phase with its tempting quick fixes. It's easy to slide back to old ways since the mind hasn't completely dialed up enough desire for change; if it had, action would already be happening. It is an opportune time to seek professional support.

Preparation: You gathered information—bought the shoes and narrowed your search for a gym. Now you are waiting for Monday to start. Beware of paradigms becoming agitated and fighting back as you attempt to launch out of your comfort zone. You may be tempted to eat your last supper, and then Monday comes and your gym clothes continue to hang on the new treadmill. Start simple and build confidence, allowing your subconscious mind to opt-in. Walk outside for ten minutes one way so you're forced to walk ten minutes back. Build more stamina as you go. Be wary of the risks of perfectionism, which sound like, "I didn't know where to start exercising," or "I don't want to start a diet until I've started my exercise routine." These statements can be forms of plan and delay. Start with walking; it is easy, inexpensive, and functional. Avoid waiting for Monday because that can turn into the next Monday, then New Year's and next New Year's, and waiting to get ready to get ready. Make progress not perfection!

Action: You made it. Your confidence is building. Measure and reward your successes. Stay accountable with a calendar or workout partner, or rescue a dog to accompany you. Pedometers and technology are also available. Journal your thoughts, feelings, and sleep patterns, and measure your successes beyond the scale.

Maintenance: You've been active for six months, and therefore, in maintenance. You built new habits with a newer mindset. You might even feel unusual if you miss a day of activity. You rarely use willpower, but more so, feel empowered to stay the course as part of your daily prescription. Avoid the risk of monotony by ensuring variety, seasonal changes, and trying new things.

The Sum of It: Listen closely to your language. You can see which phase you're in and strategize when to be gentle and/or try anew. Even Olympic athletes rest. Try an 80/20 rule by hitting the mark 80 percent and allowing a 20 percent margin for life events.

TURNING ADVERSITY INTO YOUR UNIVERSITY

I like the words of Gay Hendricks, a renowned author and psychologist, who said, "An airplane flying from Los Angeles to Honolulu will drift to the left and right the entire time it flies, but it will land in Honolulu." Although the course is set, the plane will fail many times along the way.

However, the nimble corrective system will provide corrections.

I wanted to be a flight attendant. The concept of being paid to travel intrigued me. Upon graduating from high school, I received two simultaneous blows. The school held a fashion show fundraiser for our graduation. My friends auditioned for it, so I did too. I was told in stereo, "You are too short." That week, I also learned you had to be five-foot three to be a flight attendant for most airlines, and I was vetoed twice in one week for being four-foot ten. Disheartened, I plastered a fake smile on my face and endured the fashion show. But deciding on a new career choice was more than I could grit my teeth through at the time.

I wasn't academically strong. In fact, I was placed in the special needs class. I was slow to learn, slow to read, and passed my classes by the skin of my teeth! My mother worked at the school, so she would overhear teachers talking about students in the lunchroom. One day, she came home looking sad—I happened to be the student the teachers were talking about that day. Mom tried to spare me, but I extracted what she heard. One of the teachers had said, "Karie won't amount to anything." Mom consoled me, despite my inability to console her. The memory eventually faded, but unbeknownst to me, I internalized the narrative of that conversation as my dialogue. I convinced myself to take a backseat on career endeavors, thinking, *What's the point in trying?*

A few years passed and the memories faded into my tapestry until I experienced a flashback, ironically, while sitting on an airplane. I watched the attendant reach and cram an oversized carry-on into the overhead compartment while I sat excited to reach my destination—backpacking Down Under. I could see the truth. I could never reach those bins, after all. I was, indeed, too short to be a flight attendant, and, in my glee at embarking on a six-month journey, a wave of joy rushed over me. I was proud of my new adventure, with a new direction, and that I had caught the memory of not amounting to much sitting on that plane. As the plane lifted off, I left it all behind. My grip on the past loosened, and I discovered my university in my adversity.

> "Every adversity, every failure, and every heartache carries with it the seed of an equivalent or greater benefit."
>
> — Napoleon Hill

A COURSE IN TRANSFORMATION

When you were younger, you probably couldn't wait to be older, and when you were older, you likely wanted to be younger. You and I are always looking for a change, but we fear it at the same time. Without change, you and I might not be here. Through change, you become your own hero, though it may not seem it at the time. Similar to the stages of change discussed above, *The Hero's Journey* by Joseph Campbell and *A Course in Miracles* suggest there are phases in transformation too. I've attempted to combine them below, with notes on the inevitable paradigms you face as you near success.

1. **Undoing:** You realize something isn't right and change is needed. Your heartburn/weight is connected to excessive meal portions, "wing Wednesdays," and late-night snacks. Sacrificing these can create a sense of remorse, but your symptoms are getting your attention.

2. **Intuition Is Calling:** A nudge calls you to a higher purpose and/or

optimal health. Refusing to jump in, you vacillate between wanting to change and wanting to remain the same, but the call becomes louder as it tries to lead you to the next phase.

3. **Sorting:** You start making changes and notice benefits. When you slip and fall, the feelings, good or bad, intensify. You fear sacrifice, and more events and temptations come to test you even more. However, negative feelings keep nudging your positive changes. You begin to find compromises, like trying fish tacos instead.

4. **Relinquishment:** Awakening to feeling so much better, you let go of the feeling of sacrifice, knowing the rewards are beginning to outweigh the sacrifices. Your late-night coffee isn't worth the insomnia after experiencing good sleep. You cross a threshold and others begin to notice and express interest, wanting to join you. You were the brave one, inspiring them to grow. You seem to have new support and resources to help keep you going.

5. **Settling Down:** You are more at peace, with minimal upheaval and quicker recovery from a fall. You welcome new ways. Old ways lose their grip, and only the people who matter, matter.

6. **Achievement:** You reap the rewards of rising out of adversity into your university. You see the school of hard knocks was there to teach you so you could carve a path you would not have seen otherwise. Your mess has become your message and you arrive at a place of acceptance and achievement.

All in all, there are phases in change, and knowing that may take the pressures out of not getting to your goal fast enough. Less guilt, less pressure may mean more successes.

REFLECTIONS

1. Think about a change you experienced and the stages of change you went through from denial on. What allowed you to continue?

   _____

   _____

   _____

   _____

2. What adversity became your university? What adversity is still waiting?

   _____

   _____

   _____

   _____

ACTION STEP

What exercises can you implement for one week? List the days, the duration, and time of day you will begin. Take one step, like walking for ten minutes in one direction. You will have walked for twenty minutes when you get back.

SUMMARY

You are no longer boxed into your current circumstances, nor are you defined by your past. You do not need to be held captive by your hurt. You get to choose. Everyone falls, but some things cannot rise without a fall. The victim rising to victory is the true hero, and movies are often based on this archetype. Be the star of your own movie. You get to choose yourself. Like the airplane, you can implement a nimble system to correct for the winds and deviations along the way. Learn a new language and find support—change is inevitable, and for that, you can be grateful. Arguing for anything different is futile.

> "Arguing with a fool proves there are two."
>
> — Doris M. Smith

AFFIRMATION

I take imperfect action with support, knowing only the people who matter really matter.

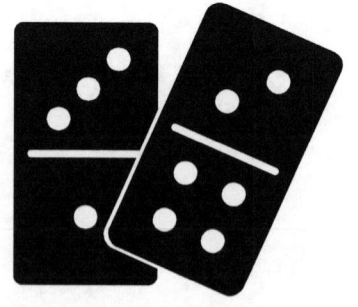

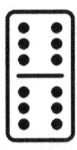

CHAPTER 12

WHAT DO VEGGIES AND FORGIVENESS HAVE IN COMMON?

"I never knew how strong I was until I had to forgive someone who wasn't sorry and accept an apology I never received."

— Unknown

Who hasn't experienced resentment? From hormones to digestion, emotions can create disease. Anger and stress hormones like cortisol can increase cholesterol, blood pressure, blood sugars, acid reflux, chronic fatigue, etc. Dale Carnegie once said, "Our fatigue is often caused not by work, but by worry, frustration, and resentment."

Think about resentment. Does your breathing become constricted? Most pay little attention to their own health while digesting resentment. The bandage of caffeine or antacids is an easier reach than purer remedies for resentment. Some conceal their resentment and become "people pleasers." I personally went from shy to "tiny but tough." I was so good at the tough act that it no longer felt like an act anymore. How about you?

My tough act was from fear of being hurt again, but I came off like a porcupine to keep people from coming close. My trust issues fueled my tough side while internalizing my shy, vulnerable side when I felt susceptible to perpetrators. Does this sound familiar? Danger may be an illusion, but the stress that illusion causes hurts us anyway. The victim-me looked to place blame, but doing so resolved nothing, leaving this "tough cookie" a pile of dough. Then a small voice inside me said, "What if you are to blame? What are you afraid of? I thought you were tough?" In that pivotal moment, I realized I needed to change; I was suffocating myself. As this quote from an unknown author poignantly said, "Change is not easy, but remaining in a constant state of grief and resentment is harder."

A Course in Miracles says, "Forgiveness is a block in perception that removes a block in me to see love's presence." Once again, it came down to the basic emotions of fear and love. Fear disguised itself as tough to protect me from love. I was blocking love's presence. I thought going inward was the best thing I could do. When I finally took responsibility, I wished I had done so long before. My life started to turn around. I had more energy, slept better, and so on. They say holding on to hurt/resentment is like drinking poison—you end up hurt, and the one you resent goes on with their life. *They* (whoever they are) are right.

I didn't know it at the time, but I reverse-engineered the Domino Diet Formula. I started recognizing the results of one battle after another. My results were caused by my actions, how I dealt with my feelings. My anger directly correlated with my fight-flight hormones being in overdrive. My breathing was shallow and constricted.

Of course, this was all a byproduct of my negative thinking. The thing is: I didn't know where the thinking came from. *What do I need to forgive so badly?* I wondered. By that point, being angry was just part of my character; therefore, I didn't even know what to go looking for. My childhood trauma would rise sometimes, but I believed being aware of it without streaming tears meant I had dealt with it. Turns out, pent-up, undealt-with hurt doesn't work that way. It requires a process of forgiveness.

Forgiveness is like vegetables—like it or not, it is good for you. Forgiving doesn't mean condoning hurtful behavior, but loosening your grip, allowing you to move forward. Chances are the other person doesn't even know they take up real estate in your mind. In the end, you benefit by making room for what really matters.

Your dream is in the land of love. If you are in the land of hostility, your frequency does not match your dream. When you release and heal, the dream becomes reachable. Much like consuming vegetables, you benefit from inner healing. In both cases, you will renew. Though I was afraid to forgive and "let them off the hook," it was me who was off the hook when I did.

BITTERSWEET: BEING BITTER OR BETTER

"No matter how much you visit the past, there's nothing new to see."

— Unknown

An elderly couple walked through the hospital doors. As they walked down the hall, I suddenly recognized them. Like a volcano building with molten lava, memories began to flood my mind. I wanted validation and a confrontation with *them* now! If I'd had a mountaintop, I would have shouted, "I deserve more than your denial for the anguish I experienced from your son! *He* robbed me of my childhood." I hadn't even comprehended that I had this gaping wound or how far down into its crevasses I had fallen.

Now, standing in the hall a few feet away, my tiny but tough fists clenched as I marched toward them with heavy stomps—as opposed to my usual clicking of heels. I wanted each step to reverberate with my point. My stride was speedy compared to their frail shuffle, giving me little time to plot the encounter. I remember thinking I could spin around and lock eyes long enough for them to recognize me and then reap the benefits of their sympathy.

Instead, I turned, and before our head-on collision, I became a deer in the headlights. I gazed into their eyes and could see frailty and sadness. Time moved in slow motion long enough for me to remember they were in a hospital, after all. Of course, they had sad eyes—there's not a lot of joy in most hospitals.

Regardless, they didn't recognize me. In a flicker, I went from "It's all about me" to "I wonder if they are grieving too." Instantly, a calm washed through me as though I had drank a magic potion diluting the poison of my resentment. The potion was called *compassion*, and although it tasted bittersweet, I felt the resentment leave me.

The definition of atonement is: Reparation for a wrong or making amends. I experienced atonement that day, and so can you.

DOUBLE-DIPPING

Forgiving someone is one thing, but forgiving yourself is another. It is the same formula, but sometimes you need some "double-dipping." When you think of someone who hurt you, you tend to hyper-focus on the situation. When it comes to yourself, though, you have a record of *all* your mistakes and punishment too. Often when we make mistakes, we gather them all together in a stacking effect, as though there were no self-improvement between them. Plus, have you ever caught yourself holding onto guilt, convincing yourself it's heartless to let go too soon? What if holding onto resentment baggage is correlated to weight gain baggage? I suspect if the link was understood, there would be a lot of baggage dropped off to be filled with atonement.

Being able to forgive my childhood demons put me on a whole new level, allowing me to see differently and receive reciprocal forgiveness myself. From there, I could see lessons and learn from them or stay in bitterness. Acceptance allowed me to stretch even further in an exercise of finding twenty good memories, despite the hurt in my past. The amazing thing was the benefits were two-fold. The hurt from me or done to me carried the same message. Things like mistakes can help you hone your intuition to know better next time. It taught me about judgment, and it made me wiser in raising my daughter. I have a connection to and compassion for others with a similar story I would not have had otherwise. I am familiar with how unknown, suppressed feelings morph, how they degrade your thinking and health, and how to help extract them. I received a double dose of forgiveness in that lesson and so will you!

SPEAKING FOR LOVE OR EATING FOR FEAR

The tiny but tough character I developed appeared to serve me, but truthfully, if healing took place instead, with proper communication tools, the resentment may not have built and I wouldn't have had to act tough in the first place. Sound familiar? This goes for the people pleasers and so on, too. The relevance goes beyond the masquerade being uncovered, again; it is about the niche of this book: health. When you don't speak it, you might find your resolve instead by eating your hurt, anger, or resentment. It took years before I learned tools such as the Angry Iceberg, spearheaded by John and Julie Gottman. Their research describes anger as the tip of the iceberg. If you remember our friend Steve, who befriended Jack and Daniels, that's all he knew how to express. Underneath, though, was fear, pain, exhaustion, loneliness, embarrassment, and so on. Not knowing how to let his guard down, he spewed anger instead, leading to arguments and defensiveness. Consider, though, if he had removed his armor and allowed himself to be vulnerable, his compassion may have been reciprocated in his relationships. This is a much better remedy than bypassing emotions and feeding addictions.

According to Mat Boggs, of the Brave Thinking Institute and author of *Project Everlasting*, in long-lasting marriages, "conflict is neutral." Furthermore, Gay Hendricks, author of *The Big Leap*, says, "Most couples have not had hundreds of arguments; they've had the same argument hundreds of times." If the inevitable conflicts in relationships were handled kindly, using communication tools, pressure, stress, and disease just might improve. Is it such a stretch to think heart disease could be related and/or emotional eating may be connected? Assuming there is a connection, below are tools adopted by Mat Boggs to improve communication.

Boundaries for a Fair Fight:

1. No name-calling.
2. No labeling. "You're just like your father/mother."
3. No sarcasm. "Oh, you are so trying, yeah right."
4. No silent treatments instead of talking things out.
5. No hitting below the belt—pushing "sensitive buttons."
6. No bringing up the past—building a case for your point of view doesn't solve the issue.
7. No "always/never"—absolutes like these undermine progress and are highly unlikely to be true.

What about past conflicts or current missteps where you could catch yourself in the midst of an error in judgment by saying, "Can I have a do-over? I'm not happy with how I handled that." Gay Hendricks and Mat Boggs also suggest the Ten-Minute Sweaty Conversation as outlined below.

The Ten-Minute Sweaty Conversation:

1. Set the intention: "I would like to have a ten-minute conversation; is now a good time? My intention is to grow and be better with you."
2. Here's what I see: Tone down the emotion; stick to facts. "I see a pattern in our conflicts."
3. This is how I feel: "I'm getting scared I will lose you when you drive away in the middle of a disagreement." Feelings will have a word such as sad, mad, or overwhelmed. Do not say, "You made me feel." No one can make you feel; you decide how you feel based on your thoughts. It's an inside job.

4. Here's what I would love: "When conflict arises, and you need to leave, I would feel less scared knowing (with my thoughts) you are coming back in a reasonable short while that allows you to cool and me to feel less abandoned."
5. What would you love? "I'm not sure how much time I will need to cool off, but we can try thirty minutes to start."
6. A new agreement: "I agree to give you space for thirty minutes so we can have a healthier conversation and help us grow."

What happens when you go too far and realize you are at fault? An apology that comes with, "I'm sorry but…" isn't an apology. Mary Morrissey suggests using the following perfect apology formula.

The Perfect Apology Formula:

1. Here's what happened: "I didn't express my true feelings."
2. Take Responsibility: "I allowed stress to build, and my anger wasn't fair to you."
3. Here's what I am doing to fix it: "I am learning ways to manage stress."
4. Here's my plan to keep it from happening again.

Note: When using the above conversation tools, don't forget to take calming breaths.

> "Never forget the nine most important words in any family—I love you, you are beautiful, please forgive me."
>
> — H. Jackson Brown, Jr.

REFLECTIONS

1. Reflect on a situation that required forgiveness. List twenty positive outcomes that resulted from that situation.

   _____   _____
   _____   _____
   _____   _____
   _____   _____
   _____   _____
   _____   _____
   _____   _____
   _____   _____
   _____   _____
   _____   _____

2. What diseases are you risking by holding onto anger, hurt, resentment? How does hanging onto your feelings serve you, and who benefits if you let them go?

   _____
   _____
   _____
   _____

ACTION STEP

Reaping the Benefits of Healing: When you notice feelings of resentment or unforgiveness, repeat the affirmation below five times. Place a note where you brush your teeth, on your shower, on your door, on your desk, or in your vehicle to remind you of what to do when resentment rises. You remove everyday tartar buildup, so do the same with any negative emotional buildup—rinse and repeat with forgiveness. It might be needed daily. Don't forget to include forgiving yourself.

I forgive you completely.
I free you from our past.
I accept healing now.

SUMMARY

I devoted an entire chapter to forgiveness, conflict, and communication tools—it is that important. Like vegetables, forgiveness' benefits are worth it even when it seems to taste bitter. Healing comes from the inside, and as long as you are breathing, you and others will make mistakes. Relationships are preordained, and so are stress-induced conflicts, hurts, and fears. Forgiveness, apologies, healthy communication, and boundaries are for your benefit in the end. Buried feelings can morph from uneasiness to addiction to disease. Reciting a forgiveness affirmation is worth it for the release; as Vonda McDermott Certified Life Coach says, it's not a one and done, but a daily rinse and repeat soul-cleansing. More than helping with your diet, healthy relationships are here to teach love and provide a mirror for you to see yourself while shining a light on self-love.

"Put down the flashlight; pick up the mirror."

— Gay Hendricks

AFFIRMATION

I release all negativity. I am not my past. I am not my body. *I am love!*

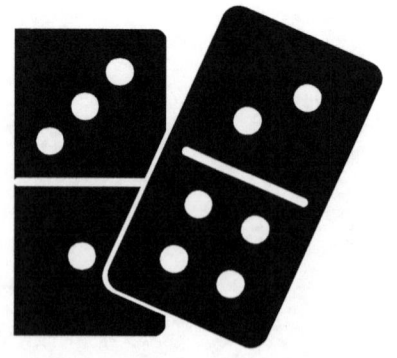

SECTION 6

THE FIFTH DOMINO—STEPPING INTO YOUR AUTHENTIC YOU

The Domino Diet Formula: Action

Thoughts⇒ Breath⇒ Hormones⇒ Feelings⇒ **Actions**⇒ Results⇒ Freedom

---

"The first year it sleeps, the second year it creeps, the fifth year it leaps."

— Unknown

Did you know the bamboo tree, despite its eventual height, only grows a few inches a year in the first five years? A little sprout appears, but to the naked eye, it may not look worthy of growth at all. If you had your heart set on seeing a bamboo tree by your measure of progress, you would be incredibly disappointed. On the other hand, understanding the evolution of this magnificent tree, you would know that the wait is worth it. Later, it will produce exponential growth, topping out at upwards of eighteen feet!

John Boggs, CEO of the Brave Thinking Institute, suggests you are like the bamboo tree. While bamboo sprouts appear minimal on the surface, underneath, root structures called rhizomes are building. The large rhizomes are essential to providing support for the ultimate height of your tree and to weather the storms. What appeared small and unworthy on the surface may, underneath, be the most significant. How you measure your wellness success matters. Spend the time patiently understanding your evolution while nourishing your body, managing your cravings, banishing body shaming, and building a stronger foundation because you, too, are building rhizomes. Is having resilience and longevity to withstand storms worth the wait?

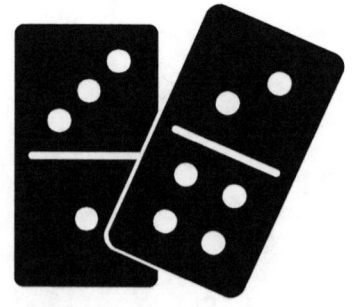

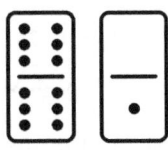

CHAPTER 13

UNCOVERING CRAVINGS

"If hunger is not the problem, then eating is not the solution."

— Unknown

You are hardwired to survive. In the distant past, your entire day from dawn to dusk would have been based on the search for food. Your subconscious wants a full belly for as long as possible as often as possible. Therefore, fat, sugar, and salt have an advantage over salads. You just finished a heavy late supper, but you still crave chocolate. You snack in a flurry while cooking supper because it was of the utmost importance to endure centuries of feast or famine. There is a tug-o-war with sacrifices on diets while surrounded by abundance. It's a paradox, really. Unfortunately, marketing schemes speak to the outdated psyche, persuading you to forgo healthy eating and stock up on two for one boxes of cookies instead. If you are still reading, you're a trendsetter, grooming new territory, no longer berating your cravings, but understanding them and their healthier rhizomes.

> "Do not go where the path may lead; go instead where there is no path and leave a trail."
>
> — Ralph Waldo Emerson

Why do you have cravings? You learned earlier about triggers and associations with food such as movies and popcorn. Less obvious still are cravings associated with the fear of hunger. Your body, along with the 7.8 billion others living on the planet, requires fuel. Yet restrictive diets often ignite hunger. When you choose a restrictive diet, your conscious mind (5 percent) is working against your subconscious mind's (95 percent) search for food. As I mentioned earlier, what many call a plateau in weight loss is highly attributed to your subconscious assessing and altering your internal situation, adjusting the rhizomes and the tree growth, if you will. If it deems it necessary, the subconscious alerts your systems to search for food, and at the same time, lowers your metabolism to preserve energy.

Understanding your subconscious, your DNA, is a new territory when operating calmly within abundance.

Just a generation ago, your parents/grandparents experienced different times, and from the different levels of thinking inherent to their situation, they passed their fear of lack down to you. They had good intentions, being completely unaccustomed to the abundance of today. How could they have taught you to navigate portion distortion when they were rationing. They were saying, "Eat everything on your plate; there are starving children in the world." This comes from their earlier brush with starvation.

The stocking up for a rainy day mindset has made us susceptible to deals like four bags of chips at $2.50 each. Subliminally, you might fall for the bargain from a mindset of supply. But do the math; it's not a bargain. You just spend more and need more willpower to overcome your cravings in your well-stocked home.

If you learn your body's signs and signals when it's guarding your metabolism on behalf of your survival, you can better customize your own calorie needs and health goals. For example, your height, weight, movement, and age are unique and far removed from the one-size-fits-all diets being pushed on the masses. With a nourishment mindset, you can monitor yourself for headaches, lethargy, shaky hands, lack of concentration, insomnia, panic attacks, dizziness, and cold symptoms as a sign you are not eating enough. As the body attempts to preserve energy and fat stores, it will take everything it can from your limbs by switching on your fight-flight hormones to keep your internal organs functioning. It is no wonder panic and binge episodes happen! Your cravings are clues. Understand them. Work with them. They are there for a reason.

BREAKFAST TO BREAK-THE-FAST

Building a solid foundation for your day starts when you rise in the morning. Let's look at the morning (or whatever time you wake as a shift worker). After fasting all night, it is time to *break the fast* (breakfast). Fueling your system properly can help you avoid cravings later. Hunger in the morning was normal as a child, but many adults have little to no appetite for breakfast. Over time, many ignore hunger cues as almost being a nuisance or flaw. Instead, you may fill up on coffee, staving off what would be normally increasing hunger. Meanwhile, your metabolism compensates by slowing systems, and you feel more fatigue from the lack of fuel and your adjusting metabolism. While in this conservation state, you might try to fight the increasing fatigue with more caffeine. Momentum builds as your subconscious remains on alert, still needing calories and nourishment. At the same time, the caffeine can lead to dehydration, which also increases hunger cues. By late afternoon, you are nearly exhausted and your cravings increase. The vending machine's candy and high-sugar beverages seem like a good idea! You may be triggered and *not be thinking* about apples.

Leaving work at the end of the day on an empty tank can set you up for even more cravings. Imagine you pick up the kids on the way home. They remind you to grab milk. Where is milk in most grocery stores? How strong are you walking to the back of the store with kids trailing behind, smells wafting from the deli, and chips, chocolate, and ice cream gazing back at you? How about the fast-food restaurants lining your way home, and with the kids plucking at your heartstrings too? If you manage to dodge those bullets, when you get home, you are even hungrier. Do you gorge from the pantry while cooking dinner? The handfuls of crackers and cheese become 300-500 calories before your main meal.

Hunger overall can switch you into fight-flight and create different choices when grocery shopping or ordering off menus, or even in the speed at which you eat. Be it a conscious or unconscious choice to restrict eating, the consequences can be similar. Your cravings are there to help you survive, and in the long run, staving off cravings can lead to portion distortion, as odds are you won't be craving a huge salad.

However, evening cravings are seldom due to hunger since most people are still digesting supper. Still, you may be low in overall nutrients. How will you know if your craving is legit? Try experimenting with a small breakfast and pay attention to your cravings through the day. Many notice fewer cravings even by evening simply by having sustenance as far back as the morning as a result. Certainly, the subconscious might be content with sufficient fuel. Find compromises using the conscious mind to make small changes and become proactive about cravings. You may also find the craving checklist below helpful.

CRAVING CHECKLIST

- **Sweets:** This could mean low sugar symptoms (poor concentration, headaches, mood swings, being clumsy). Has it been more than three or four hours since your last meal? Are you low in carbohydrate fuel? Try a small apple and one tablespoon of peanut butter or half a cup of trail mix or half a cup of flavored yogurt. We'll talk more about carbohydrates, etc. in the next chapter.

- **Salt:** Could be dehydration (slight hunger, headaches, brain fog, darker color urine, poor coordination) caused by excessive sweating, alcohol, caffeine, or high blood sugars. Stay hydrated. Try one cup of vegetable soup, crackers and cheese, or pea pods and hummus.

- **Chocolate:** This craving may result from altering hormones during menstrual cycles, sleep disruption, stress, and/or craving serotonin. Go for a walk while listening to music. If the craving is still there, try strawberries dipped in chocolate pudding, one cup of hot chocolate, or one or two squares of high-quality chocolate.

Note: For recurring cravings, look for patterns/timing. Assess for possible nutritional deficiencies by discussing your cravings with your doctor and/or dietitian. See my website for more (www.TheDominoDiet.com).

UNI-TASKING

When you think of addiction, substances like alcohol probably come to mind, but there are other addictions. The first step in the Alcoholics Anonymous Twelve-Step program is admitting you have a problem. You cannot overcome something you're unaware of. Do you have an addiction? In this discussion on cravings, my intention is to present a mix of addictions and cravings that often remain under the radar.

Earlier, I discussed the dynamics of eating while watching the news or skating across the floor to the dishwasher and igniting the fight-flight hormones while digesting. Eating fast creates a kind of amnesia where you forget you actually already ate until your indigestion reminds you and where things like gluten are blamed instead. From a solutions perspective, though, mealtimes that are held sacred, with an allotted duration and mindfulness (plus minding your fullness), provide better absorption of nutrients and allow for balanced meals with proper intake volume, which would perhaps help avoid triggering cravings.

Renee was a bank manager who, when it came time to raise kids, put her career on hold. A few years into being at home, she got an invitation to her high school reunion, which would be nine months later. She was intrigued but embarrassed by her seventy-five-pound weight gain. Her husband suggested seeing a dietitian, but she declined, saying without conviction, "I'm too busy."

Renee had everything planned, with meals, lists, and chores highlighted on sticky notes. However, time for herself hardly made the list. Truthfully, her planning addiction kept her distracted from something else. It was clear she was easily overwhelmed when her routine changed. In fact, the idea of hopping a flight to the reunion made her so anxious she deleted the email invitation altogether. Oddly enough, while she was driving her son to hockey, he asked to see a dietitian for sports nutrition like a friend had, and Renee immediately agreed. Then something clicked—when it came to the kids, she was willing to adjust anything and everything. Something else occurred to her at that moment—part of her hesitation in going to the reunion was her concern the kids would eat unhealthily all weekend. She even thought losing weight would mean buying new clothes for herself instead of the kids. She was a martyr in disguise, which was more about control, since her own weight was out of control in her opinion, and she was hiding her fear. Somewhere in the heap of distractions and sticky notes, Renee lost focus on herself and placed it on everyone else.

Renee knew during her pregnancies that eating healthy was manageable. With that in mind, she decided it was time for her new birth—and just in time for the reunion, too.

Renee began working with her dietitian for her family to take small steps together. The kids learned chores and became more self-sufficient. Renee had once thought that even if she delegated, she would end up having to do *it* anyway, but now she realized this belief was a symptom of her perfectionism, and coddling her kids was not helping anyone.

Renee started walking during her son's hockey practice and she would eat/fuel more often throughout the day—she had been notorious before for skipping meals. Here is where we circle back to cravings and learn from Renee; previously when she ate, it was on the fly while multitasking under stress. Her corresponding stress was a potential culprit in her weight gain. Her calorie intake was so low during the day that her craving increased at night. However, she justified those cravings with another version of "I hardly ate. I was too busy." Working with her dietitian, she started uni-tasking at meals, pausing and slowing down. She immediately noticed she had less indigestion and more energy. It occurred to Renee that slowing down to enjoy meals came with the fear of uncontrolled eating. When she calmed herself, however, the opposite happened. In reviewing her food journal, she noted the highest nighttime calorie intake correlated with earlier skipped meals.

Renee managed to be sixty pounds lighter when she hopped a plane to her reunion, and she continues to make progress today. Beyond her weight change, she admits the best part is, "The person I became in the process." Her addiction to being busy was a coverup for fear of losing her sense of purpose after giving up a career and losing herself. Being the perfect wife and mom gave her purpose and something to control while her identity eroded. That changed when she understood what she was really craving.

Once Renee gained confidence and renewed health, she continued to put the oxygen mask on herself first, and she felt fulfillment in her days. Even better, she connected with an old friend at the reunion, and together, they started an online business from home! Something as simple as slowing down, uni-tasking, and pausing to eat and seeking support created a domino effect in the right direction.

What are you craving besides food?

REFLECTIONS

1. What cravings do you have most and when? Do you skip meals?

   _____

   _____

   _____

2. Do you take time to enjoy your meals? Do you multitask during meals, and if so, why? Does it save you time in the end? What about your health?

   _____

   _____

   _____

ACTION STEP

Experiment with a *pause* before meals. Be mindful of what, how, and where you are eating and take the time to eat without distraction. Use a sticky note to remind you of your sacred time and to enjoy it.

Power of the Pause Prescription: Take three times a day and/or as needed!

P-ause before eating.
A-ware of breath (breathing in through the nose, out through the mouth).
U-ni-task, mindful eating, remove all distractions.
S-low down; let your stomach and brain work to signal when to stop.
E-njoy with love, guilt-free.

SUMMARY

Some of your cravings may be related to scarcity thinking. Abundance surrounds you, though. Create a sacred time to slow down while mindfully enjoying meals. Fuel throughout the day, keeping cravings at bay and break-the-fast with a nutritious meal each morning. Then you will no longer be swayed by marketing because you will be an abundance trendsetter. Your rhizomes are built, your sprouts are growing, and you are ready for a new growth too.

AFFIRMATION

I have all the time required to R&R and nourish myself at meals and throughout my day.

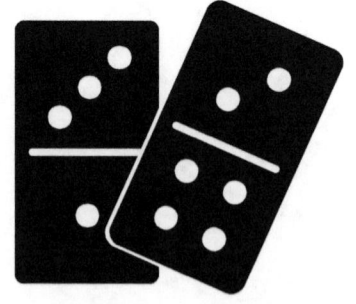

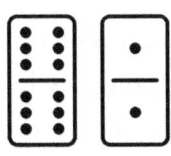

CHAPTER 14

BANISHING BODY SHAME AND THE HUNGER GAME

> "Judging a person does not define who they are; it defines who you are."
>
> — Wayne Dyer

Would you finally like to love yourself unconditionally? Do you feel judged? Do food relationships and body shame control you? When you love yourself, are you more compassionate and less judgmental of yourself and others?

Sarah was a beautiful, vibrant twenty-year-old who had inherited her mother Gwen's long, thick hair and bright-blue eyes. However, Gwen, despite her beauty, lamented her pear-shaped body. Gwen became a chronic dieter, which affected the entire household. Before family occasions, Gwen, in fear of judgment, would be triggered to frantically try on clothes with her husband running around trying to appease her with accolades. He wanted to go, Gwen wanted to stay, and Sarah was left watching a game of ping-pong she had to tiptoe around. The following day would start another dieting cycle for Gwen, complete with the anxiety of Monday morning judgment when she stepped on the bathroom scale. The whole household was on a rollercoaster.

Sarah couldn't understand her mother's plight. She would sit watching Gwen as she applied makeup, enamored by her mother's beauty. Sitting with her mother, Sarah became somewhat like a priest taking Gwen's confession as she pointed out her own flaws and sins (food battles). The word sin is a Greek term meaning "miss the mark." Seanna Quinn, certified yoga instructor and wellness coach, suggests, "The subconscious tracks and listens when you miss the mark, looking and speaking of your flaws looking in the mirror. [This] can leave mental pictures you carry around while creating a feedback loop you see even more while hyper-focused on them. All this while airbrushed images, wrinkle creams, control tops, fake eyelashes suggest you aren't good enough the way you are."

Unfortunately, Sarah inherited more than her mother's beauty. At age fifteen, she developed body dysmorphia (severe body image distortion). Vowing it would only be the one time, she stuck her finger down her throat. Her vow was soon broken again and again, on top of obsessive calorie counting and exercise. Her mother soon noticed Sarah's thinning hair and a callus on her index finger. Gwen knew the signs of malnutrition from anorexia due to the loss of her sister, who had battled anorexia growing up. All the red flags were there: baggy clothes, yellowed skin, brittle nails, and three months with no menstrual cycle. At first, Sarah blamed the issue on stress, but soon Gwen knew it was time they both sought help.

With the aid of a support team, Sarah and Gwen developed a new relationship with food. They were able to see the nourishment and fuel side of food. They chose the healthy mind to body approach over the societal approach. Together, they encouraged and congratulated one another. Their subconscious minds paid close attention. They healed together, and a door opened for Sarah to build a career in nutrition while closing the door on the bathroom scale and dieting cycles.

I have always admired how vulnerable and brave Gwen was in recognizing they both needed help. She showed herself to be strong in seeing her contribution to the problem and her ability to be a part of the solution too. Coming together in support was key for mother and daughter!

BALANCING THE SCALES

"The measure of success is not whether you have a tough problem to deal with, but whether it is still the same problem you had last year."

— John Foster Dulles

Rob joined a gym intending to build lean mass and lose weight. He hired a dietitian to help put a plan together to reduce calories while ensuring adequate nutrition and endurance to actively build muscle. Rob's past attempts had failed after two or three weeks for two reasons: 1) Low energy/stamina, and 2) The scale stayed the same. From his perspective, the results were not worth it. His dietitian explained the problem of obsessive weighing and the reality of weight and muscle shifts. She advised him to avoid weighing himself for three or four weeks. After two weeks of diligently sticking to his healthy lifestyle, his friends insisted on taking him out for dinner and drinks, which led to late-night nachos and beer and two days of missed workouts. Despite Rob's promise not to, he weighed himself and noted he had gained four pounds. He contemplated giving up, as per the usual two-week threshold, even though he was feeling healthy overall. He called his dietitian, who told him it may not be true weight gain.

You are worth more than your weight on a scale, and your weight is worth more than you think. Ligaments, bones, muscle, and fluid all weigh on the scale. The average sixty-four-kilogram (140 pound) woman and seventy-seven-kilogram (170 pounds) man have 7.75 kilograms and 11.5 kilograms bone mass, respectively. Plus, you contain an average of 70 percent water, 30-45 percent muscle, and 7.75 percent blood volume.

The rollercoaster of weighing in can be exhausting and frustrating, offering dreadful feedback despite your efforts. If you went to your boss daily after working hard and got berated despite your efforts, what would happen to your motivation to continue? Weighing in on a scale has so many variables and hyper-focusing on the scale provides an incomplete evaluation of your progress. For instance, pound for pound, muscle and fat weigh the same but take up different space. Rob may have put on muscle, which the scale also reflects. Without measuring inches, his evaluation was inadequate, especially since gaining one pound of muscle can burn an extra twenty-five calories an hour while sitting. Your metabolism increases with more muscle. The benefits of building muscle far outweigh the scale.

Inaccurate interpretation of scales has created obsessions and distorted food relationships with foods pitted against foods. In fact, some diets suggest removing foods that have been around for centuries. Fruits that nourished your ancestors are now, suddenly, after thousands of years treated as forbidden because of their sugar content. What? The generation of portion distortion wants to lay blame on fruit or the gluten in grains? Is it the ten grams of sugar (two teaspoons) in one cup of fruit or the sixty grams of sugar (twelve teaspoons) in a twenty-ounce juice to blame? Is it the three teaspoons equivalent of sugar in one slice of bread or the ten to twelve teaspoon equivalent in a large muffin? Plus, fruits are rich in antioxidants to help fight diseases like cancer, and the fiber in grains has a host of other benefits. Sadly, numbers on a scale have become more important than effective strategies to fight cancer and other diseases! Overall, eating disorders are rising to epidemic proportions, and "disordered eating" occurs at an even higher advancing level. They share similar symptoms with disordered thinking at the root but to varying degrees, as shown below.

Anorexia and Bulimia Symptoms:

- Purging or use of diet pills and laxatives
- Obsession with food, calories, and dieting
- Changes in mood and emotional state
- Distorted body image (dysmorphia)
- Hormone changes noted with missed cycles or lost muscle
- Excessive exercise
- Denial of hunger and refusal of food
- Engaging in food rituals
- Chronic weighing
- Always on a new diet
- Avoiding restaurants and family occasions

Do these symptoms sound familiar? Suffice it to say, society measures progress by numbers, grades, IQs, bank accounts, years married, age, height, and of course, weight. What about your mental health? Where are the numbers for measuring it? What if your health progress was measured differently and offered rewards? Would you stay the course? The little sprouts that grow in health, like sustaining or increasing energy, endurance, strength, fewer headaches, mood swings, or depression are the rhizome measures of your true success. Does your weight define happiness or is it the other way around? It's time to make your diet a way of life.

TRADING YO-YOS FOR DOMINOS

> "There is no diet that will do what eating healthy does."
>
> — Unknown

Mémère (Grandma) reached for a warm cinnamon bun and sheepishly announced, "I'll go on my diet again on Monday." I was perplexed while looking at Mémère, who was nearly seventy-five years old. I remember thinking, *Weight loss is still a concern for you?* I was young and not yet a dietitian, but I instinctively knew the diets she spoke of were not positive. I wanted Mémère to be free and cut herself loose from the chains of vanity.

As I discussed earlier, extremely low calorie diets can cause hormonal imbalances and be a breeding ground for malnutrition. Anything under 1,200 calories, as most diet programs are, has the potential for nutritional deficiency. Plus, there isn't a one-size-fits-all calorie count—

and your calorie needs differ from day to day. Most women need more than 1,200 calories a day, let alone men. Still, the dangling carrot of losing weight despite possible muscle breakdown remains a lure.

How do you know if your diet is unhealthy? If weight release is too quick (more than two pounds per week), it often reflects muscle or water loss. Low energy, headaches, dizziness, depression, hair loss, irregular heart rate, brittle nails, and/or frequent illnesses are also clues. Water loss is common in the beginning of diets, especially because they limit salt and processed foods. Also note that water retention during the menstrual cycles can swing weight upwards of five pounds. A true one-pound weight increase requires an intake of 3,500 calories above your basal metabolic needs.

Further, weight change often comes with an adjustment period called a plateau. Think of when you change time zones or adjust to daylight savings time—it takes a few days for your circadian rhythm to recalibrate. The same goes for your metabolism. When you release weight, the subconscious might try to find it again, causing a yo-yo diet effect. If you want to release and set weight free, work with the inevitable plateaus and trade the yo-yos for dominos. Using your understanding of the subconscious to gauge your tiredness and the other clues mentioned above, make slow adjustments to calories according to your body's needs. You may need a rest day or more recovery time too.

Change your activities from time to time and avoid the all-or-nothing trap. Focus on fueling your day by ingesting proper nutrients and know that cutting back further on calories doesn't always work. Despite how counterintuitive this sounds, you may need to increase your calorie intake. When you make a change, track your intake for two or three days and report to your dietitian to help adjust your plan. Your dietitian will likely suggest a calorie range for active and nonactive days as a wiser concept instead of a fixed calorie approach. You do not live in a fixed world, right? Slow and steady with slight modifications to intake and activity as shown below may be more viable.

Walking:
20-30 mins burns ~ 150-200 cal x 30 days = ~ 3,500 cal (1 lb)

Reducing in Diet:
~ 150 cal x 30 days ~ 3,500 cal (1 lb)

Total Release:
~ 2 lbs a month x 12 months = 24 lbs (sustainable)

Not having second helpings could deduct between 300 and 500 calories. Walk briskly for one hour and you could burn 300 to 500 calories. Try ten minutes of brisk walking to burn about 100 calories, which adds up to a ten-pound release in one year. However, the reverse is also true. For instance, a glass of wine at 100 to 150 calories over time can add up to a ten-pound weight gain. Below are examples of calories in common foods.

Examples of 100-150 calories	**Examples of 500+ calories**
1 oz of cheese	2 slices of pizza
1 cup of juice	2 cans of soda
2 tsp of fat (butter/oil/margarine)	4 tbsp cream salad dressing
1-2 wings	1 chicken burger
6-8 oz wine	16-20 oz wine
1 baked potato	1 large order of fries

3 cups of popcorn	1 small bag of chips
10 almonds	1 cup almonds
1-2 mini chocolate bars	1 average size chocolate bar
12 nacho chips with salsa	20 movie theater nachos with cheese

PORTION DISTORTION

> "To eat is a necessity, but to eat intelligently is an art."
>
> — François de La Rochefoucauld

Two squirrels, Pat and Parker, lived near Banff, Alberta, in the tall trees. They actively gathered food and nesting supplies every day, but one day, a delicious smell from a nearby restaurant wafted by Pat, who became intrigued. Pat moved curiously toward the aroma and stumbled upon a feast in a large metal bin. With a full belly, Pat went home and fell into a deep slumber. Meanwhile, Parker remained busy gathering supplies. When Pat woke, the bin called, offering another buffet. This routine continued as Pat lost the enthusiasm for staying active. The associated weight increase was hard on the joints and made moving difficult. Listlessness set in, so Pat decided to ease the load by moving next to the restaurant bin. Confessing to Parker, Pat offered to share the bin, but Parker declined. Pat, with less mobility, developed more aches and pains and slipped into depression. Luckily, Parker visited, knowing what to do to get Pat back on track, and with that, they reunited in the woods where Pat returned to a healthier way of life and was completely renewed.

You and I come from times of feast and famine, but today, famines are rare and have become feasts or super-sized feasts. Food volumes are increasing while mobility decreases. Juice, for instance, used to be in small, plastic, half-cup containers (125 milliliters). Today, juice and soda are in sixteen- to-twenty-four-ounce individual portions! How many oranges does it take to fill one cup (eight ounces)? How about twenty-four ounces? What would happen if you ate ten oranges? Liquid calories are underestimated; i.e., black coffee has little to no calories, but with the added cream and/or sugar, it can increase to 200 to 500 calories a day. This daily habit can add up to 250 calories in no time. Why pick on nourishing food like fruit compared to empty calories (meaning they contain calories without the nutrients in others).

Whether you eat at home or in restaurants like Pat, supersizing can occur. Most meals have about 500 to 700 calories, and with second helpings, about 1,000 calories. This is where most weight increases come from.

In a study of 1,000 participants, group one made no lifestyle changes while group two consumed less processed food and walked for thirty minutes a day. Group two, after the lifestyle changes, lost fat and experienced 70 percent less disease over a ten-year span. Yet, this isn't news to most. Still worthy of noting, though, is how subtle these changes were.

Compromises can be another subtle approach to lifestyle changes and can save calories and allow you to enjoy your favorite foods too. A large bag of chips with 800 calories could instead become one cup added to three cups plain popcorn. Your snack would then be 300 calories, saving 500 calories, and therefore, a potential 3,500 calories (one pound) in one week. See the illustration below.

Walk 45 mins: = 500 cal x 7 days a week = 3500 cal = 1 lb.

Meal or snack: -500 cal x 7 days a week = 3500 cal = 1 lb.

Tracking intake using apps or a calorie counter can help you develop an understanding of calories since even healthy foods like almonds add up (one cup is about 500 calories). Use these tools as learning devices to adjust your habits, but avoid the obsessions they can create. The calorie counter below is also a quick way to assess your plate.

Simple Calorie Counter Table:

Grains	½ cup = 70 cal
Veggies	½ cup = 5-40 cal
Fruit:	½ cup = 45 cal
Milk	½ cup = 40-90 cal
Protein	1 oz = 25-70 cal
Fat	1 tsp = 45 cal

Average Calories for Weight Release with Moderate Activity

	Male:	**Female:**
Breakfast	400-500 cal	300-350 cal
Lunch:	400-550 cal	350-400 cal
Supper:	600-700 cal	400-500 cal
Snacks	100-200 cal	100-150 cal
Total:	**1700-2000 cal**	**1350-1700 cal**

* The above are estimates. Refer to my website for ways to customize your calories (www.TheDominoDiet.com).

LEARNING TO HAND JIVE

For portion control, you can also try a smaller plate, thereby automatically lowering calories, fat, salt, and sugar. Dividing your plate into half vegetables and the remainder divided equally between grains and protein can help. Or try the "hand jive." You have a tool you can take everywhere that is customized just for you. Your hands! Your hands match your stature with your fist being equivalent to one serving of fruit, potatoes, vegetables, cooked grains, and so on customized for you. In some cases, like pasta, which is less dense compared to rice, one or two fist-size portions on active days is reasonable. Eating palm-sized portions of meat, chicken, or fish at most meals works. Your thumb equals one serving of cheese, dressing, or peanut butter. Feel free to use *handfuls* of vegetables when you are extra hungry. The hand jive works for kids too.

HUNGER HELPER

As discussed earlier, fear of hunger runs deep. Ironically, despite the abundance of food today, fear of hunger plays out through your day, often unnoticed. Statements like, "I'm eating so I won't be hungry later" or marketing ploys like .50¢ more for super-sized meals are misguided. The biological aspects of hunger and belief statements such as, "I'm not eating all day so I can feast tonight," don't work. Where did this thinking even come from? Deep-rooted fears of hunger from your subconscious arguing for your survival will hold more water than this myth. Your conscious mind can decipher and measure your hunger to help navigate hunger pains, but more so to keep the fight-flight panic overreaction at bay. With your conscious mind, you can ask, "How hungry am I, and what's the panic?" To help optimally fuel your metabolism, try the hunger scale below.

Hunger Helper Scale: 1-10

1—I'm full and digesting my last meal. If I am thinking about food, I'm triggered!

2—I'm not hungry. I'm not full and still digesting my last meal.

3—I'm getting tired. Not hungry yet. Time for hydration.

4—I'm a little hungry; mealtime is in a couple of hours. Time for a snack and water.

5—It's close to mealtime. I can wait until then to eat; a little water won't hurt.

6—I'm getting hungry; time to prepare my meal, calmly.

7—I'm hungry; time to eat before my eyes become bigger than my stomach.

8—I'm eating, and if I'm not careful, I risk eating too fast and too much.

9—I'm eating and have to ask myself to slow down.

10—I'm starving and out of control. Calm down; it's not my last supper!

* If you are not hungry in the morning, assess your night snack (more discussion ahead).

Hunger Helper Food/Beverages

You assessed your hunger, and although it's unexplainable, you are legitimately hungry but still want to stay true to your goals. Maybe you're on your way to the restaurant and want to avoid overeating. In any case, below are healthy choices to fill the gap with free snacks—low calorie foods loaded with nutrients. All vegetables are low calorie, but a few are virtually calorie-free. Browse the list below for appealing win-win choices.

* Try tomatoes sprinkled with your favorite herb; drizzle with balsamic vinegar.
* Create a stir-fry or antipasto cooked in broth; drizzle with lemon/lime, herbs, or garlic.
* Water, tea, low sodium broth soups, sparkling water

Asparagus, Broccoli, Cabbage, Cauliflower, Celery, Cucumber, Lettuce, Mushroom, Onions, Garlic, Peppers, Radish, Spinach, Tomato, Zucchini, Salsa, Kale

THE EATER'S DIGEST: MORNING STARTS AT NIGHT

Did you enjoy a bowl of cereal before bed as a kid? Did your grandparents have toast and tea with the evening news? Why now, after years, is a nighttime snack considered bad? There are more rules on when or when not to eat, what to eat and not to eat, than ever before, and yet obesity is still increasing. Rules like do not eat after 8:00 p.m. come with a misunderstanding of food digestion. Writing a rule book without understanding digestion is misguided. For instance, if you eat a light dinner and then play basketball, getting back home at 8:30 p.m., do you simply not eat? One of the most important teachings in sports nutrition is to have a recovery snack post-workout. In fact, I've always said your best workout starts with your after-workout nutrition. What if you consume a healthy salad at 5:30 p.m. and are hungry at 9:00 p.m.? Do you criticize yourself or have a snack? Many children have nighttime snacks to help them sleep. Much like the recovery snack, the nighttime snack may be where your best morning starts. Does this sound controversial? It is possible the problem lies in the difference between snacks and snack meals.

Understanding food digestion can help you better plan various work shifts, tournaments, eating on the road, etc. Overall, a good rule is to eat small, frequent meals, starting with breakfast. As I mentioned earlier, if you are a shift worker, your first meal is still break-the-fast time, although it may not be morning. Start with something even if you have no appetite. Otherwise, having your largest meal at breakfast is worth a try. You might notice smaller meals follow quite naturally. Studies show grazing and/or eating every two to three hours can help manage blood sugars, cholesterol, high blood pressure, acid reflux, and more. Your body can manage foods in smaller amounts. Additionally, if you go longer than three or four hours without fuel, you could be setting yourself up for cravings. Below is a reference on food digestion variables to help you plan small meals.

I will explain the role of carbohydrates (carbs), protein, and fat in the next chapter. For now, let's focus on digestion. Carbohydrates can take anywhere from five to ninety minutes to digest. Juice, soda, sugar, honey, and hard candies enter your stomach, digest, and move into your bloodstream within about five minutes. As easily digestible fuels, quick-release sugars won't stave off hunger for long but can help with hypoglycemic (low sugar) episodes and/or in fueling athletes, but excessive sugar is often stored as fat.

Other carbs such as whole fruits take about thirty minutes to digest, while yogurt, pudding, and smoothies take about forty-five to sixty minutes. A slice of white bread takes about sixty minutes, while high-fiber foods (more than five grams of fiber per serving) digest in about ninety minutes. Protein fills you up, taking about two to three hours to digest. Lean protein like skinless chicken can take about two hours to digest, but with skin, it takes about three hours because fat takes about three to five hours. Combined foods, such as bread and peanut butter, can lengthen digestion time as do extra-large portions. See digestion times below.

Carbohydrates: five to ninety minutes (higher fiber, about ninety minutes)
Protein: two to three hours
Fat: three to five hours

Overall, consuming small, frequent meals with carbs, protein, and fat can provide more nutrients and leave you feeling satisfied. Consuming fat or protein without carbs can fill you up but not fuel you as carbs are designed to do. On the other hand, carbs alone can cause sugars to rise. In the end, watching your portions and eating smaller, more frequent meals or snacks and combined foods like apples and nut butter is wisest. In truth, nighttime snacks from the past were not the problem, but how they morphed into super-sized meals with some of the highest calorie counts of the day is. Sadly, the nighttime snack gone wrong has ruined it for many, especially if you normally chose nourishing snacks. With diabetes, for instance, blood sugars are often better managed with small, frequent meals, including carb and protein combined snacks. Those with high morning sugars often note improvement with a proper evening snack also (discuss with your dietitian). Heavy snacks, though, can increase sugars. Understanding food digestion and interpreting symptoms can help you gauge and adjust your snack for a good night's sleep, and therefore, your morning does start at night. See the indicators for snack changes below.

Heavy Snack: reflux, nightmares, stomach cramps, thirst from salt, skipping meals.

Insufficient Snack: restless legs, insomnia, fatigue, headaches, portion distortion.

Nighttime snacks can now be determined by the hunger scale and realistic monitoring of symptoms, portion control, digestion times, and activities and be customized to your needs. Suggesting no snack doesn't work because it remains an Achilles' heel for most. Compromises, however, often work. The next few chapters will provide more information, but for now, bring back your cereal or toast and nut butter for a light, two- to-three-hour digest. The fiber can keep you satisfied and the nutrients, like calcium and potassium, can often help prevent leg cramping. A small wrap with peanut butter and banana is a great recovery snack for muscle growth after physical exertion or check my website (www.TheDominoDiet.com) for more ideas and recipes. Below are more healthy snack options.

100-150 Calorie Snack Choices:

- 1 Serving (½ cup) all Fruits and Vegetables (1 cup for most vegetables)
- ½ Baked Potato with 2 Tbsp Salsa or Cottage Cheese or Light Sour Cream
- 1 Cup Soup (hearty) 2 cups Broth-Based Soup
- 1 Slice of Bread/Toast
- 1 Cup Cereal
- ½ of 1 Cereal Bar
- 1 Mini Brownie
- 1 Mini Muffin
- 1 Tbsp Nut Butter
- ¼ Cup Nuts
- ½ Cup Edamame Beans
- ¼ -½ Avocado
- 2-3 Tbsp Hummus

- 1 Egg
- 1 Mini tin of Flavored Tuna
- ½ Cup Yogurt/Cottage Cheese/Pudding/Ice Cream
- 1 oz Cheese
- 6 Cups of Popcorn (no fat) 3 cups popped in oil
- 2 tsp Butter/Margarine (add to popcorn or use cooking spray or hot sauce for seasoning)
- 2 Cookies (cream-filled)
- 3-4 Plain Cookies (small)
- 4-6 Crackers
- 30 Pretzel Sticks
- ½ Cup Salsa
- ½ Cup Chips (12-18 chips)
- ½ Popsicle
- 1 Cup Regular Hot Chocolate
- 1-2 Squares Chocolate/Mini Chocolate Bar

*Note: The calories above are averages. It isn't about counting calories so much as being aware of the above to strategize your meals and snacks for a fueled day.

DOMINO DIET MOMENTS

Unfulfilled Thoughts⇒Fight-Flight⇒Hungry⇒Portion Distortion ⇒Stuffed⇒Sluggish

Mindful⇒Pause/R&R⇒Fulfilled⇒Portion Control⇒Satisfied⇒Fueled & Nourished

REFLECTIONS

1. Achieving optimal health requires steps. List three to five steps you can start with.

   _____

   _____

   _____

   _____

   _____

2. What meal patterns can you change to make your diet a way of life?

   _____

   _____

   _____

   _____

3. List some of the ways you can measure your overall health progress.

   _____

   _____

   _____

   _____

ACTION STEP

Use the hunger scale while monitoring your portion changes. Try a small plate and three meals and two or three snacks a day, noting your satiety, energy, and sleep while adjusting your meal and snack plans along the way to match your goals.

SUMMARY

Measure your results with a new mindset, guilt-free and without a bathroom scale. Banish body shaming for good and set yourself free. You are more than a number, especially considering your overall vitality. Clearly, pressure diets and their yo-yo effect risk damaging your metabolism. Consider a slow, steady approach, without scarcity or lack thinking, and keep your favorite foods with a little portion control. You can determine through compromise what you are really hungry for and customize what you eat, and then your healthy mind can help the dominos fall from "Mind to Micronutrients" to your health freedom.

AFFIRMATION

Chin up, beautiful. You are not struggling; you are simply mid-conquer!

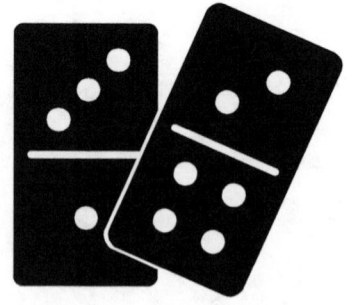

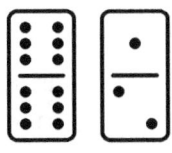

CHAPTER 15

YOUR FOUNDATION

"You can't build a great building on a weak foundation."

— Unknown

One morning, four burly men attempted to put together a new plastic shed. They gathered all the pieces and placed the written instructions aside. They thought using the picture diagram would be quicker. After a few hours of assembly, frustrations arose because the walls were not aligning with the floor. Improvising, they forced the alignment, with each man squeezing the walls just enough to allow a rod to thread through the ready-made holes. The rod could now hold the roof in place. This would also allow the adjoining walls to shift into place for the screws to thread and the bolts to hold everything in together. Before completion, it was time for a much-needed break; they left the extra supports with nuts and bolts to be the last part of the project.

As the men quenched their thirst, a sudden *Crash! Bang!* boomed in the background. Like private detectives, they dashed to the crime scene. The small rod, doing its best to hold things together, had completely sheared under the pressure, causing all four walls to collapse. It was time to refer to the instructions. There it was in bold print: "You need to build on a level foundation." They had not.

Is your eating plan built on a level foundation? What instructions do you follow? Plant-based, vegetarian, Keto, Mediterranean? Does your meal plan adjoin to all of your needs, your schedule, etc.? While searching the internet for information on diets, you may feel overwhelmed by the inconsistencies. One article promotes more protein while another advocates for higher carbs with a vegetarian diet. Unless you understand how to distinguish your nourishment needs, you could end up "collapsing" energetically too. You require a level foundation to withstand the underpinnings of pressure. Certainly, crash diets promising ten pounds off in one week so you can squeeze into your dress are makeshift ways that can leave you unsupported.

WHOLLY MACROS

Consuming adequate calories in your diet (your way of life) is your level foundation. Inadequate or too many calories can create challenging results. You also need four walls for a solid structure, albeit unique to your size. Macronutrients—carbohydrates, protein, fat, and water—are like four walls. To eliminate a macronutrient is like removing a wall. Although water does not have calories, the other three macronutrients do, and their calorie content is listed below. Also worth mentioning is alcohol (which is not a macro) because it also contains calories, as indicated.

Carbohydrates: 4 cal/gram

Protein: 4 cal/gram
Fat: 9 cal/gram
Alcohol: 7 cal/gram

Let's look at each macronutrient now in more detail.

Carbohydrates: Carbohydrates are usually separated into *simple sugars* (sugar, honey, syrup, jam, candies) that are low fiber and easy to digest, and *complex* sugars (fruit, vegetables, grains, legumes) that are high fiber and take longer to digest. Dairy products, such as yogurt and milk, are a carbohydrate source since they contain lactose (sugar). Pastries and other baked goods contain sucrose, so they are also carbohydrates. Although not all carbohydrates are equal, gram for gram, their calories are equal to those of protein. Yet, the weight industry, where calories matter most, battle between proteins and carbohydrates in this last decade. Following a low carb diet can have risks because most carbs, in fact all macros, are intrinsic in disease management. Why, then, do carbs have a reputation for being "bad"? There are, indeed, healthy and not-so-healthy choices, but the same can be said for fats and protein. Still, carbs are the most efficient source of fuel for your body; your brain alone requires about 120g a day. That is equivalent to 2 slices of bread, 1 cup of rice, 2 fruits, 1 cup of milk, and 2 cups of vegetables. Combined, they would equal about 600-700 calories, which is still extremely low. Your specific carbohydrate requirements vary according to activity, age, sex, etc. On average, women require 200-250g and men require 250-300g or 45-50 percent of their total calories per day to be carbohydrates.

Protein: Protein can be found in plant (legumes, nuts, and grains) or animal (meat, fish, poultry, eggs, and dairy) sources. It is absorbed differently from carbohydrates. Protein is needed for the growth and repair of muscle, plus many hormone and cellular developments. It can also be used for fuel, but not as efficiently. From sitting to bodybuilding, your daily needs can vary. Most people require 1g per kilogram of *ideal* body weight or 20 percent of total calories. Notice the keyword is ideal body weight. Some have misunderstood this calculation as 1g per pound. That calculation would almost double the protein total. Consuming more than you require will result in the extra being stored as fat, not muscle. In fact, excessive protein, according to some studies, can compromise those susceptible to renal (kidney) disorders. Then again, too much of anything can have negative consequences.

Fat: Fat is essential for healing, lubricating joints, cell membranes, skin, hair nourishment, and more. Although fat is the highest in calories of the macros, the daily requirement is lower. On average, 20-30 percent of your calories should come from healthy fats or approximately 40-60g per day for women and 60-80g per day for men. Examples of healthy fats are fats are olive, nuts, canola, and flax oil. Fish oils rich in omegas are also encouraged. Note, the cholesterol in healthy fats varies from no cholesterol in plant sources to higher levels in animal sources because cholesterol is made in the liver. No liver, no cholesterol. Egg yolks are a high source of cholesterol, but egg whites have none. Consuming 3-4 eggs a week is considered safe if you have higher cholesterol levels and one egg a day if there are no known Heart Health risks. In many Heart Health and Weight Management programs, using healthy fats in moderation is encouraged due to the calories. Note: Most fats that are hard at room temperature (butter, lard, and some margarines) are called saturated fats and should be used sparingly.

Alcohol: Alcohol is higher in calories than protein or carbohydrates but rarely considered in calorie calculations despite its association with weight gain. Some studies suggest red wine can lower blood pressure and increase good cholesterol (HDL), but the counter to this is an estimated 700-1,000 calories in a bottle of wine, which incidentally, is the same for a six-pack of beer. The overall benefit or risk of alcohol requires a case-by-case assessment, but the general safety limit for alcohol is one or two drinks per day as indicated below.

Alcohol—One drink equivalent examples (100-150 calories)
Five ounces of wine, red or white
Twelve ounces of beer
An ounce and a half of liquor

DRINKING WATER WORKS

The often-overlooked macronutrient in your diet is water. Water is a conduit for cells, hormones, and for circulation, joints, eliminating waste, etc. You are 70 percent water, but this isn't a one-time volume. You are constantly using that reserve and in a continual need of replenishing it. Neglect to hydrate and you risk becoming like a stale pond. The more salt or sugar you consume, the more hydrating you also need. Caffeine and alcohol, albeit liquids, can be dehydrating. To replenish, most suggest six to eight eight-ounce cups of water a day. But you can customize your intake using your own barometer. The color of urine is a useful indicator: clear meaning hydrated and darker yellow meaning you are not! You don't love water? The following tips can help.

1. **Fresh or frozen fruit:** Enhance your water with lemons, limes, oranges, berries, watermelon, or cucumber slices, which also add nutrients.
2. **Bubble Up:** Buy or make your own sparkling water with plenty of flavor options or use ginger, mint, or cold-brewed herb tea.

3. **Icy Cold:** Studies show you will drink more when water is ice cold. Try flavored ice cubes or frozen fruit.
4. **Drink Tea:** Try herbal, fruit, green, white, caffeine-free teas. Have black or green teas earlier in the day, and try chamomile tea at night for better sleep.

JAVA JUNCTION

Not everyone has the same tolerance for caffeine, and your tolerance can change with age and hormones. An empty stomach can also increase the jitters and ignite low sugars, especially when your coffee masks your hunger temporarily. Monitor your tolerance to determine the effects on your sleep and/or anxiety. You may need to take your last sip approximately five to six hours before bed or earlier, which is how long caffeine lasts in the body. Still, coffee isn't the only source of caffeine. A forty-ounce container of soda or a twelve-ounce iced mocha or energy drink has more than 300 milligrams of caffeine. Teas vary in caffeine content with caffeine-free options. Some products and medications have hidden caffeine, i.e., the herb guarana. What are your caffeine limits?

Caffeine Limits: about 300 to 400 milligrams per day for adults; 300 during pregnancy; 80-100 for children.

Caffeine Content of Popular Drinks:

Energy Drinks: 100-400
Espresso: 100-150
Coffee/Tea: 80-100
Soda: 40-60

Chocolate: 30-100

* Measurements are milligrams per cup (250 milliliters); 50-100 grams of chocolate.

* Pregnancy: Some teas like raspberry leaves can induce labor. See your doctor/dietitian.

IT'S NOT PASTA'S FAULT

For centuries rice, bread, and pasta were staples. Suddenly, in the last twenty years, they are in question. Grandma spent hours in the kitchen making bread, serving roast beef, potatoes, carrots, and homemade pie. According to today's measures, she was poisoning us with gluten, red meat, and sugar. Really?

Only in North America is pasta served as a meal with powdered cheese. Italy serves pasta as a side dish. The two are not the same, and yet pasta has the bad rap for causing weight gain. Is it pasta's fault? In the '90s, type two diabetes and heart disease were primarily diagnosed in elderly populations. Today, children are at risk. Once upon a time, morbid obesity was rare, but now more categories have been created to make room for extreme morbid obesity. Clearly, diets restricting pasta and other carbohydrates are not working against these trends.

What if positive relationships with food along with stress management occurred instead and attention was placed not just on what you eat, but on what you are not eating? With the abundant food supply in First World countries, we risk being overnourished with some foods but undernourished with others. Did you know consuming four or five servings of fruit and/or vegetables a day can lower most cancer risks by 40 percent? Yet there are cries about the sugar content in fruit. Is the concern of cancer not worth the sugar in fruits Mother Nature provided for nourishment? Eat low carb is a broad statement. Fruits and vegetables are carbohydrates rich in antioxidants and fiber. Since when is it a good idea to lower fiber or antioxidants in your diet when, in fact, you may need more? Is it the teaspoon of sugar in your coffee or honey in your tea, or is it the five teaspoons of sugar and cream in your five cups of coffee? Maybe it isn't about the potato but the huge bag of chips? The pasta or the rice alone are not the only problem, but what you pour on them might be. Don't forget, fat has more calories overall. If you stick to quality over quantity and leave room for vegetables, you can perhaps enjoy your pasta with a glass of wine too.

"Our minds, like our stomachs, are whetted by the change of food."

— Quintilian

Tip: If you love pasta, try making dishes with a higher ratio of vegetables like tortellini, ravioli, or penne pasta added to a Greek salad. When in Rome, eat pasta as a side dish.

* Tomato paste/sauce is rich in lycopene, an antioxidant linked to lowering risks to heart health and certain cancers. Load with peppers, carrots, zucchini, or mushrooms!

* Try spaghetti squash and tomato sauce for twice the veggies and double the nutrients.

DOMINO DIET MOMENTS

Scarcity/Lack ⇒ Fight-Flight ⇒ Unlevel Foundation ⇒ Susceptible ⇒ Disease

Healthy Thoughts ⇒ R&R ⇒ Nourished ⇒ Resilient ⇒ Vital Whole Health ⇒ Harmony

REFLECTIONS

1. What diets have you followed, be they low-carb or low-fat? What did you experience? What caused you to stop following it?

   _____

   _____

   _____

   _____

2. Have you experienced dehydration? What are the signs your body gives you?

   _____

   _____

   _____

   _____

ACTION STEP

Do you have a solid foundation? Spend the next two to three days monitoring your hydration, energy, and sleep patterns. Is caffeine doubling as a dehydrator and sleep depriver? Pay attention to the signs of dehydration. Try focusing on monitoring your hydration levels as a goal for the week, and purchase several water bottles you can distribute in your home, office, and vehicle to remind you to drink more fluids. Then monitor your benefits.

SUMMARY

Eating is a requirement; it isn't just a luxury. Not everyone has the same needs, which vary with size gender, activity, and even healing needs. Your style, preferences, and culture should be reflected in your eating plan much like your own unique home. Your calorie needs are specific to you, and the same can be said for your macronutrients. Assessing your calories for two to three days can give you a balanced assessment. Remember, though, alcohol contains calories and can also be dehydrating. Therefore, make water the gold standard beverage overall. As well, it isn't about taking away caffeine, but more so, being mindful of the amount in relation to your tolerance and your precious sleep. Is it the carbohydrate, protein, or fat, or is it the amount relative to your needs? What do you put in your coffee/tea…daily?

"Thousands have lived without love, not one without water."

— W. H. Auden

Tip: Set a colorful box of flavored herb tea on your desk/counter to catch your eye and replace coffee later in the day.

AFFIRMATION

Every day, I am aligned, stronger, healthier, and happier.

* Please note the numbers in this chapter were based on overall averages. Refer to my website (www.TheDominoDiet.com) for ways to personalize your nutritional needs measurements.

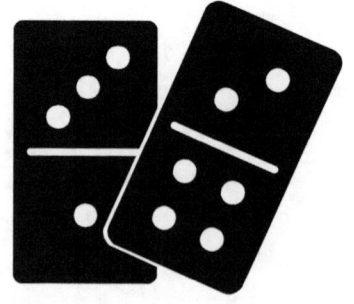

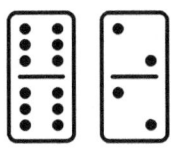

CHAPTER 16

ARMING UP WITH MICRONUTRIENTS

"Nutrition is the only remedy that can bring full recovery and can be used with any treatment. Remember, food is our best medicine!

— Bernard Jensen

I thought it was normal. I was thirteen, reading the *Nutritional Almanac* like it was *Vogue* magazine. Over three decades, I witnessed each macronutrient (macros) take its turn as the good or bad guy. During the '80s, bodybuilders obsessed over carbs with "Carb-Up" powders in demand. Protein powders were in plain packages like brown sugar is today. They were chalky in texture and hard to mix, never mind the taste. Amino acids were in demand but not seen as the building blocks of protein they truly are. Fructose (fruit sugar) hit the market running and marketers proudly boasted formulated recipes containing it. In fact, many recipes suggested using fructose as a better natural sweetener. The word natural was all the rave too. A bias in perception, though, since table sugar (sucrose) is from sugarcane and, therefore, obviously natural too.

By the '90s, the focus was on fats. Carbohydrates were still okay but no longer held the spotlight in the era of lite beer and diet sodas. In the '90s, lengthy grocery shopping with a detective badge in hand was the norm. Selections of cold-pressed oils (olive oil, peanut, flax, etc.) were sought after, plus margarine replaced butter, lard, and shortenings. You needed to compare products or be deceived. For example, some "lite" hot chocolates contained the same calories and sugar as regular, but lite referred to the container volume, which was the same price. Overall, new trends meant new confusion.

In the 2000s, protein was the attention-getter, pushing fats to the back and axing carbs. The push for protein focused on making you feel fuller and weight loss. However, the Western diet was hardly low in protein in the first place. Did I miss something? Meat has been a staple for years. With heart disease on the rise, heart health guidelines suggest smaller meat portions and more fish, fruits, and veggies, but instead, the hype suggested carbs are evil, especially fructose. Do you see a pattern? Promote one and create mass confusion with another and cycle through the macros to find something new to promote. Yet each of the macros has benefits, and to suggest otherwise means part of the equation is missed and/or a lack of understanding. For one, there is a hidden army of nutrients in macros to be brought to the frontlines.

FLEXITARIAN

What if you were ahead of marketing that is playing to the naïve? Maybe a flexitarian diet can be your next trend? Meat occasionally, fish more often, and meatless days too. It does not have to be all or nothing. Why such mass confusion on the path to true health? Adjust portions rather than eliminate foods, and voila, you can have pasta, potatoes, or rice sharing a plate with protein and vegetables and still be fine.

I want to reach out and extend my apologies to you. It has been a frustrating ride, to say the least. Who can you trust, and how can you keep up with all the fads? It's time to end the battle and focus on whole foods with carbs, protein, fat, and water united by shopping the perimeter of grocery stores—fruits and vegetables, grains, meat and other proteins, and the dairy aisle ring the outside of grocery stores. You can still make room for more. It's a matter of ratios. A positive relationship with food can return too. If true health is the mission and anyone wants to stake their claim, it is best to know the whole picture. While the macro goliaths were pitted against each other, the hidden army was forgotten. The Davids against the Goliaths if you will. In fact, I trained as a dietitian with the International Olympic Committee. According to another David I met during that time, including all macros and micros to fine-tune performance can make the difference in the rise from novice to elite athletes. This David went from dragging across the finish line in pain to being a qualifier for Team USA and the Goliath of World Championships, simply by arming up with all the macros and micros. David Dixon states, "I was restricting my diet of carbohydrates due to mixed messages, but by following a Flexitarian way of eating, I recover quickly, perform better, and feel healthier. I found a way to put the heal back into my health by listening to the needs of my body with the mind in lead." Let's now peel the layers back and put the heal back into health.

"You can't see the picture when you're inside the frame."

— Les Brown

PUTTING THE HEAL BACK INTO HEALTH

If whole foods filled the bulk of our shopping cart, I suspect we wouldn't feel the need for a science degree to read a label. Think of the fruit and vegetable aisle—not too many labels there, right? There are two primary reasons whole foods have been altered or replaced. Convenience and marketing. I love the convenience, too, but the price we are paying is high in more ways than one.

The reason you have access to instant foods (i.e., rice, oatmeal, and potatoes) is the demand for convenience. The fiber on a kernel of brown rice, for example, takes longer to cook. Therefore, manufacturers created fiber-stripped products to speed up the process. The labor and packaging then increase the price. You have companies who offer convenience and their marketers are making more money. Although grabbing an apple is pretty convenient, perceptions deviate with boxed and canned foods. Most of these items are carbs once rich in nutrients and fiber. It's possible carbs took the brunt of the being-stripped-down-for-convenience attack but processed foods might be the bigger problem. Ironically, now more protein is suggested to fill up what the fiber once did as a natural filler and calorie-free at that.

Studies have correlated diseases to the consumption of processed foods. With nutrients stripped and digestion and/or absorption compromised, your immune system needs even more protection. Also, the added salt, sugar, and/or fat in processed foods can be more than you bargained for. The protection we get from the *army of micronutrients (micros)* the macros contain needs the spotlight now. This is, by and large, the biggest reason I suggest embracing all macros (carbs, protein, fat, and water). They contain so much more. Carbohydrates are not only your main fuel source, but they carry most of your micros like vitamin A, B, C, calcium, zinc, potassium, fiber, antioxidants, etc. Proteins contain iron, keratin, B12, and healthy fats such as nut oils, avocados, olive, vitamin A, D, E, K, and omegas.

The moral of this story is all vitamins and minerals come from macros, and blanket statements like "Eliminate carbs from your diet" can leave you vulnerable to disease. Granted, there are healthier choices within the realm of carbs (potatoes instead of potato chips). The same can be said for proteins (fish is better than hot dogs). Unfortunately, too many diets focus on weight loss alone and don't pay attention to the risks of heart disease or cancer, which are trending upward while whole foods slide downward. Putting the *heal back into health* means a healed mindset, healthy food relationships, arm-in-arm with whole foods and all the macros with selected healthy foods!

HEALING FROM THE INSIDE OUT

> "Every single cell in the human body replaces itself over a period of seven years. That means there's not even the smallest part of you now that was part of you seven years ago."
>
> — Steven Hall

Your body is continually regenerating, renewing, and repairing. You started as a cell containing the genetics of your parents and ancestors from thousands of years ago. New cells are forming daily. As the quote above illustrates, in seven years, your body is completely renewed. Broken bones would never mend, wounds would not heal if it were not for your body regenerating. The turnover time varies for each cell. Stomach and immune system cells turn over in two to five days, whereas bone cells take two weeks. Red blood cells (RBC) have a lifespan of 120 days. When your doctor sends you for lab work to further assess your health, your RBCs are part of that assessment as indicators of health. Your circulatory system runs everywhere from head-to-toe carrying nutrients and oxygen. Given the significance of your RBCs, I will rely on them to illustrate a few valid points.

At this given moment, you have RBCs that will die today and brand-new ones to replace them. In 120 days, you will have all new RBCs running through your entire body. This all happens naturally, courtesy of your subconscious systems. What would happen if you optimized your lifestyle consciously and holistically with: 1) A Healthy Mindset, 2) Eating Healthy, 3) Exercising, 4) A Healthy Environment, and 5) Sleep Hygiene? All optimizing those cells! There are plenty of studies showing better wound healing, bone development, etc. with a healthier lifestyle. Even the membranes of your cells strengthen when consuming essential fatty acids. Healthier RBCs mean a healthier you from the inside out. I cannot emphasize this enough. Your body can renew right down to the cellular level from disease to health harmony. New habits, new cells, new aligning, falling into place like dominos from *mind to micronutrient*—this is a holistic prescription for a whole you, and it comes free with infinite refills. Below are creative ways to add more micronutrients to your day.

MICRONUTRIENT-PACKED MEALS

Breakfast:

Egg omelet-vegetables/salsa or make a larger batch to portion into muffin tins for the week.

Whole-grain bread + avocado or hummus or salsa

or

Oatmeal* + nut butter, fruit, yogurt, cinnamon, drizzle syrup or molasses

or

Smoothie-fruit, yogurt, milk/substitute, plus seed mix indicated below.

Lunch:

Mighty Micro Soup (butternut squash, broccoli, cabbage, tomato, beans, etc.)
(use low sodium veggie broth or used canned versions and add fresh veggies)
+ high fiber crackers + nut butter, tofu, or cheese

or

Noodles + vegetables, low salt broth + tofu or shrimp +sesame oil

or

Salad-spinach, vegetables, nuts, cheese, pumpkin seeds, dried/fresh fruit*
1 small nut/berry high fiber muffin

Dinner:

Leftover soup/salad + poached salmon (or other fish) + brown rice + peppers or

Quinoa or rice bowl-vegetables, tofu, cashews, peanuts, edamame beans, sauce (i.e., tzatziki or sesame oil, dressing, BBQ)—make in large batches for the week.

or

Rotisserie chicken + salad+ raw veggies + buns and homemade milkshakes + berries

* Add chia, flax, or hemp hearts to increase fiber and omegas.

Dessert Tips: baked apple, strawberries dipped in chocolate pudding, small wrap with Nutella, and fruit cut into bite-sized pieces, fruit compote on a mini brownie or angel food cake.

Note: For customized menus, portions as per your goal, refer to my website (www.TheDominoDiet.com) for ways to work with me.

MICRONUTRIENT ROBBERS

Fast food can be low in nutrients and rob you of the opportunity for a nourishing meal, not to mention the nutrients required to digest fast food. Having an empty calorie diet whereby the calories are high in unhealthy fats, sugar, and salt, but low in nutrients can rob you of fluids, strain your system, and create digestive disorders. Alcohol can be a thief in the night, especially for those under stress or healing from inflammatory conditions. In fact, with alcohol, your body processes it as though it is an intruder, and in doing so, it requires more water to flush your system, which increases the risk of dehydration and diminishing electrolytes such as potassium. Watch for headaches, knots, and/or muscle cramps as signs of dehydration and electrolyte deficiency, with or without alcohol being a factor. As well, alcohol can rob you of vitamin A and most B vitamins. In which case, you may experience altered vision, poor balance, and an anxious nervous system. Because the stomach lining, esophagus, etc. can also become inflamed, absorption of B12 and folic acid can be affected. Keep in mind, though, that immune conditions, excessive caffeine, certain medications, etc. can cause dehydration and/or inflammation too.

Tip: Try coconut water or sports drinks to hydrate and replace electrolytes.

DOMINO DIET MOMENT

Thoughts⇒Fight-Flight⇒Anxious Cravings⇒Fast-Food⇒Micro Robbers ⇒Disease

Thoughts⇒R&R⇒Calm⇒Hungry for Fuel⇒Healthy Meals⇒Healthy Body⇒Health

REFLECTIONS

1. Do you consume five servings a day (a half cup equals one serving) of fruit and/or vegetables at meals and snacks? List five ways you could add more to your day.

_____

_____

_____

2. Are you low in specific nutrients? What foods are missing from your diet?

_____

_____

_____

_____

ACTION STEP

Listed below are dinner themes to creatively add more daily micronutrients. Write your grocery list with ideas from the meals below and enjoy the compromises of flexitarian eating. For vegans or vegetarians or other specific diets, refer to my website (www.TheDominoDiet.com) for more. Consider a check-up with your doctor for lab work to best assess your health needs.

Flexitarian Dinners

Meatless Monday: portabella burgers, grilled tofu salad, mighty micro soup, cauliflower steaks, vegetable kabobs, vegetarian lasagna/moussaka, vegetable quiche, falafel in pita bread with salad, Greek salad (add quinoa/pasta), baked Brussel sprouts.

Taco Tuesday: hard or soft shell, wraps or lettuce wraps, filled with vegetables, fish, ground meat/poultry or shrimp plus salsa, tzatziki, or bruschetta. Bean burritos and veggies.

Wok Wednesday: rice, pasta, noodles, or cauliflower rice, plus vegetables and chicken, beef, shrimp, fish, or nuts, plus sweet and sour/teriyaki sauce or sesame oil and/or pineapple.

Travel Thursday: Thai, Mexican, Asian, etc., lettuce or rice wraps, lentil curries, healthy jambalaya or won ton soup with extra veg, spaghetti squash and tomato sauce.

Fab Friday: flat bread pizza (tomato sauce, veggies, lean protein, cheese) or healthy nachos (low sodium nachos and veggies, salsa, corn, beans, avocado, cheese).

Super Saturday: BBQ kabobs, sliders, veggie foil packets, or chili loaded with vegetables. Place vegetable or fruit trays on the counter for the day—in sight in mind.

Soul Sunday: roast meat/poultry/fish and grains plus two veggies and use leftovers for soup. Try a healthy turkey meatloaf with shredded veggies, salmon burgers plus veggie salad.

Tips: Do you have picky eaters in the house? Use healthy dips like tzatziki, hummus, and peanut sauce. Vegetables and fruits have similar vitamins so use more fruit if preferred. Try baked apple, healthy banana splits, or fruit cobbler.

* Turn dairy containers (yogurt, sour cream, cottage cheese) upside down on a tray in the fridge for a longer shelf life.

SUMMARY

"Never underestimate the little things." This common saying in this case is more than true. Building a better relationship with food rather than eliminating whole foods will not only fuel you but arm you to fight against diseases and illnesses. It isn't just about what not to eat, but more so, what you are not eating. It is time to put the heal back into health, nourish holistically, renewing yourself in 120 days from the inside out.

AFFIRMATION

I am flexible, nourished, and in vital dynamic health!

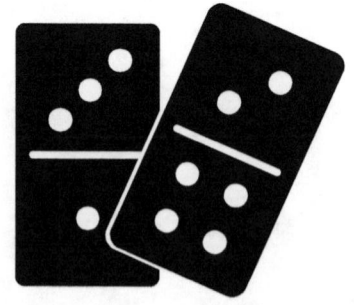

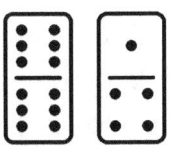

CHAPTER 17

UNDERSTANDING THE FIVE WS OF SUPPLEMENTS

"Part of being successful is about asking questions and listening to the answers."

— Thomas Berger

While I was working in alternative medicine and familiarizing myself with new shipments of supplements, it was customary for me to read the disclaimers. Labels boasted claims like, "improves memory," "energy boosting," and "speeds metabolism." I wondered how these ingredients worked in the body. I pictured these small pills and their contents from swallowing to digestion and how the body sent the nutrients marching in various directions according to their functionality. One day, a specific label stating "natural, high-potency multivitamin" caught my eye. It contained so many nutrients, like 10,000 IUs of vitamin A, 200mg of vitamin C, 100 IUs of vitamin E, and so on. I wondered how an *all-natural*, tiny, compressed pill could include so much. Like a two-year-old asking "why this and why that," I had a plethora of questions.

I had the who, what, where, when, and why questions about the supplements, to say the least! Although the word "processed" was frowned upon, how on earth were these manufactured if they were not processed? Were they synthetic? How could a bushel of strawberries and carrots being mulched, squeezed, and cooked not be considered processed? I finally called the manufacturer for clarification and was met with a long pause. Then I had even more questions with no answers.

The only answers were in the curriculum I was taught and submersed in. So many people had achieved positive results with many of the herbs and supplements I was fortunate enough to learn about. However, you don't know what you don't know. Back then, if you came to me with chronic fatigue, I advised you to take an iron supplement rather than ask about sleep, caffeine, or your diet. Then again, I didn't know what I didn't know. The combination of my alternative medicine and traditional medicine training helped with those questions. Do you have questions about supplements? Below are the common questions and answers on supplements.

Who, When, What: Some individuals require supplements due to deficiencies from a diagnosis such as iron anemia. On the flip side, a condition called Hemochromatosis requires limiting iron consumption. Folic acid (400 mcg/day) is suggested for women in childbearing years. During pregnancy, prenatal supplements are also recommended. If you are on a restricted diet or suffer from malabsorption of nutrients, and/or have digestive disorders, a multivitamin is often called for. Children may also require a children's chewable; infants often require added vitamin D drops. As well, vegetarians and vegans may require iron and vitamin B12 and possibly vitamin D, B6, and omega-3s supplementation.

Where, When, What: The sun provides vitamin D. If, however, you live in the northern hemisphere, the sun in the winter months does not offer the same absorption, especially if your skin is covered. You may want to reconsider using creams and foundations containing sunblock during these months depending on where you live (check with your doctor). In many cases, 1,000 IUs a day is appropriate but a discussion and verification through lab work is highly recommended.

How: A diet rich in healthy whole foods, inclusive of all macronutrients including milk or milk substitutes, will provide most of your nutritional needs. The exceptions are those mentioned earlier, i.e., pregnancy. Some foods have optimum absorption provided by Mother Nature. Milk, for example, is high in calcium and vitamin D, which assists in absorbing calcium. In addition, milk is alkaline (low acidity); therefore, it enhances calcium absorption. If you are lactose intolerant, this doesn't exempt you from the need for calcium and vitamin D; therefore, fortified milk substitutes are needed.

Below are common micronutrients unhealthy diets can be deficient in. Refer to my website (www.TheDominoDiet.com) for a comprehensive list of other vitamins and minerals and inquiries about learning your specific needs. Note: Dosages are specific to gender, age, and comorbidities. As well, ask about ways to enhance absorption, assist tolerance, and avoid negative interactions.

Vitamin A: skin, joints, digestion, sight, muscles, concentration, nervous system, etc. Foods: carrots, butternut squash, fish, etc. Deficiency: poor vision, dry skin.

Vitamin B: (B1 through B12) nerves, memory, muscles. Foods: protein and grains. B12 is mainly found in meat, fish, and poultry. Deficiency: mouth sores, fatigue, light-sensitive.

Vitamin C: immune system, cellular growth. Foods: fruits and vegetables and some herbs. Deficiency: poor wound healing, bruising, infections, frequent illness.

Vitamin D: nerves, hormones, bone development. Foods: fish, eggs, milk, mushrooms, and sunlight. Deficiency: weakness, osteoporosis, mild depression.

Vitamin E: heart, skin, joints. Foods: nuts, seeds, oils. Deficiency: poor flexibility/coordination or edema.

Calcium: bone and muscle health. Foods: milk products or fortified substitutes, broccoli, almonds, sesame seeds, and some greens. Deficiency: muscle spasms, osteoporosis.

Folic Acid: red blood cells, nerve cells. Foods: fortified cereals, beans, peas, oranges, greens. Deficiency: red, swollen tongue, anemia, fatigue, insomnia.

Iron: red blood cells, oxygen carrier. Foods: fortified cereals, meat, pumpkin seeds, greens, raisins. Deficiency: fatigue, hair loss, dizziness.

Magnesium: muscles, heart rhythm. Foods: grains, beans, avocado. Deficiency: irregular heartbeat, muscle cramps, irritability.

Potassium: muscles, blood pressure regulation, concentration. Food: apricots, potatoes, bananas. Deficiency: muscle cramps, reflux, irregular blood pressure.

Sodium: muscles, blood pressure regulation. Foods: processed foods containing sea salt or regular salt. Deficiency: (rare) dizziness, nausea, low blood pressure.

Sodium Guidelines: 1,500-2,000 milligrams a day (less than 200 milligrams per snack, less than 500 milligrams per meal). Excessive intake can increase blood pressure and edema (water retention).

Zinc: hormone, immune system, skin, and hair. Foods: meat, poultry, fish, oysters, nuts, seeds. Deficiency: change in taste, smell, thin nails, poor night vision.

THE ARMOR OF IRON

Melony was a fifteen-year-old, healthy athlete who excelled at Cross-Fit. After watching a documentary on vegan diets, she spoke to her parents about converting her lifestyle. They supported her wishes on the condition that should any concerns arise, she would see their physician. Melony agreed and started eating mainly fruits, nuts, quinoa, rice cakes, vegetables, hummus, and salads as quick grab-and-go items for her busy days. Since nuts are high in calories, her weight remained stable, but fatigue began to affect her endurance. Around the four-month mark, her hair started to thin and she was battling frequent colds and flu. She visited her doctor and was diagnosed with iron anemia (low iron).

Iron is available in the diet in two forms—heme and nonheme sources. The word heme means blood. The richest, most absorbed sources are heme iron from beef, pork, chicken, lamb, and fish. Nonheme sources are in plants such as leafy greens, nuts, seeds, and legumes. Melony was consuming nuts and leafy greens, but the absorption of non-heme iron is lower unless also consumed with vitamin C-rich foods (tomato sauce on pasta or strawberries in spinach salad or rice with pepper). She was advised to use a cast iron pan for preparing tomato sauce. Tomato sauce offers duel benefits because it is rich in vitamin C and acidic, and therefore, leaches iron from the pan into your sauce. Melony was also advised to incorporate raisins and iron-fortified cereal as snacks mixed with the protein from nuts. She also armored up with iron supplements. Fortunately, Melony increased her iron levels and continues to monitor them yearly.

Note: Multivitamins do not always contain adequate iron. Iron supplements are best prescribed by your doctor due to possible side effects such as liver and intestine damage. Also, with iron supplements, higher fiber meals and drinking more water may be required to avoid possible constipation. Try taking them with meals for better tolerance.

THE PROTEIN COMBO

Melony continued to learn ways to optimize her health on a vegan diet. She also discovered that plant-based protein such as nuts, grains, tofu, and legumes are absorbed less compared to meat, poultry, fish, milk, yogurt, and eggs. Plant sources are missing one or more amino acids, the building blocks of protein. Animal sources are complete proteins, containing all nine essential amino acids. The good news is that when you combine plant-based proteins, they can become complete. For example, bread and peanut butter are each missing an amino acid, but when combined, they become complete as is the case for rice plus beans and tofu or quinoa and edamame beans, etc.

GRANDMA'S PHARMACY

Grandma asked me to run to the garden for carrots, garlic, and peas. She also, with a sparkle in her eye, asked me to swing by the meadow to pick dandelions, rosehips, cranberries, and chamomile. It was a sunny morning, but the mist was still in the air, suggesting a chill. Happily, I fetched my red poncho as she looked for a basket to gather the harvest. Like Red Riding Hood, I whisked the basket from her hands and bounded down the steps toward the garden.

While I was still within earshot, she hollered, "Oh, and grab a few mushrooms near the meadow." Then nonchalantly, as though this were an everyday jaunt for me, she instructed, "But not the poisonous ones with the red caps or rings around the stems—just the white-capped mushrooms!" Although nervous, I did not want to disappoint her and carried on with the mission. I remember thinking, *Poisonous? How on earth does she even know all that?*

I returned with my basket and Grandma proceeded to inspect the harvest while separating the herbs and mushrooms. While she was preparing her dandelion salad, she began to teach me. "Dandelions are high in vitamins and good for colds."

As she tossed the leaves and yellow blossoms together, she asked me to fill a pot of water and light the gas stove. Not being accustomed to a gas stove, I anxiously grabbed the matches and went from feeling like "Red Riding Hood" to the "Big Bad Wolf" who might blow the house down, mushrooms and all. I accomplished my mission, though, and Grandma tossed the rosehips and cranberries into the boiling water.

Still teaching between humming the song "Paper Roses," she said, "Rosehips are loaded with vitamin C, cranberries are good for your kidneys, and we'll use this water later to steep chamomile tea for a good night's sleep." Grandma wasn't a nurse or herbalist; she was a homesteader with knowledge passed to her that she was passing down to me. It was quite common to use home remedies then. I remember Mémère (my other grandmother) telling me, "Molasses is high in iron and B12," as she slowly poured the black gold into her homemade baked beans. She made delicious molasses cookies too. My grandmothers normally cooked whole foods and used homemade remedies with a preventative mindset. In fact, this was a normal mindset then.

NATURE'S PANTRY

Was I naturally drawn to alternative medicine, or did it find me? Connecting the dots and looking back, maybe it was a little of both. I've been privileged to be among Aborigines in Australia, watching preparations for underground cooking (Kup-murri) and various indigenous medicinal herb remedies such as eucalyptus leaves. I was also fortunate to work in First Nation communities and speak with medicine men and women regarding their remedies and sacred secrets. They were reluctant to share their knowledge from fear it would become mass manufactured, putting their sacred plants at risk and/or tainting their medicinal properties. I was aware of how mass production can change the properties of medicinal foods, as it does with garlic.

Garlic is a well-known treatment for the immune system and heart disease. It has antimicrobial properties. However, its strong odor is a deterrent. Therefore, some companies produce odorless garlic, which involves removing allicin—one of the compounds that provides health benefits. The superior benefits of this "super botanical" are in its whole, natural form.

Herbs like ginger, fennel, dill, and chamomile are in formulas for babies with colic. Some cultures use cumin and coriander after meals to aid digestion and saffron for menstrual cramps. The list goes on, and there are plenty of books on homeopathic remedies. The point here is that there are nutrients available to you like Grandma's potions to help prevent illnesses. Today, many wait for the illness. Perhaps it is time to make room for both God's pharmacy and medical therapies, sleep hygiene, walking, and meditation. This holistic approach might be the missing link.

Suffice it to say, the more empowered your thinking, the more likely you are to make healthy choices. There may be fewer illnesses as a result! Of course, don't make changes without a risk-benefit analysis for each scenario. For example, aloe vera applied to cuts has potential benefits with low risks, if any. Cinnamon sprinkled on your oatmeal or cappuccino may help balance blood sugars, but it could cause heartburn in some. The herb foxglove contains a natural ingredient called digitalis, which is used in heart medications. Therefore, the combination of heart medications and foxglove tea may not be worth the risk.

IMMUNE-BOOSTING AGENTS

A mother's womb provides shelter for her fetus to grow with a placenta specially designed to allow certain nutrients through but keep the most harmful ones out. If you use your imagination, you can surround yourself with a veil to deflect harm and allow the good to pour through too. Placebo or otherwise, some feel it helps keep your immune system functioning at its best. Why not try—what's the harm? Why not try every angle, especially the mind, to boost your immune system? Many easily believe in the opposite. Who hasn't heard, "Flu season is here; I'll probably get it"?

You have probably heard vitamin C plays a role in enhancing your immune system. However, dosage recommendations vary with age, environment, and comorbidities. Vitamin C is water-soluble. The body will absorb what it requires and soon dispense the rest through urine. As a result, excessive doses can lead to kidney stones for some. Spreading your intake throughout the day is highly effective. One large orange can have up to 100 milligrams of vitamin C, and therefore, consuming the recommended five servings of fruits and vegetables throughout the day can easily help meet your needs. Also, foods themselves have other nutrients like fiber as an added benefit. Again, specific doses are determined better in consultation with a health professional, but a total of 500 milligrams a day of vitamin C is safe for most adults. Other known immune boosters are vitamin D, zinc, and the herb echinacea. Refer also to my website (www.TheDominoDiet.com) since each has specific dosage recommendations, tricks to enhance absorption, procedures to taper supplements instead of discontinuing any given one all at once, plus potential interactions with medications. Even something as simple as eating grapefruit can lower the effectiveness of some medications.

The other micronutrients known to enhance your immune system and help with other health conditions such as heart disease are the omega-3s found in fish. Higher levels are in salmon, tuna, halibut, trout, sardines, and mackerel. Vegans can use flax seeds, flax seed oil, or walnuts. New to some are hemp hearts, which also contain omegas and are easily added to soups, yogurt, smoothies, salads, etc.—with bonus protein too. Refer to my website for more ways to include hemp hearts in energy balls, muffins, and homemade protein bars and how to incorporate these in recovery snacks for sports nutrition.

One of the more effective, inexpensive, and often forgotten ways to help your immune system is your R&R. As I mentioned earlier, your body requires rest for healing and the R&R response can assist your immune system with calm breathing, walking, yoga, meditation, music, etc., while helping you better digest and, therefore, absorb nutrients too.

THE RISE AND FALL OF APPLES

> "Anybody can count the seeds in an apple, but nobody can count the apples in a seed."
>
> — Mary Morrissey

For thousands of years, apples have been a symbol of good and evil—from representing wisdom to Eve's curse. Sayings like, "You are the apple of my eye," "The apple doesn't fall far from the tree," and "One bad apple spoils the bunch" are part of our culture. But recently, apples have gone from "An apple a day keeps the doctor away" to "Apples have too much sugar." However, in all my years as a dietitian, weight gain or illness have rarely correlated with apple consumption, or consumption of any other fruit or vegetable for that matter. Juice, on the other hand, might be the spoiler of the bunch with its higher sugar concentrations. The whole apple with peel is high in nutrients and insoluble fiber (does not dissolve in water). Inside the apple are rich nutrients and soluble fiber (dissolves in water). Once again, consuming foods in their whole form changes how we digest them. Brown rice, legumes, and barley are high fiber but low in today's fad diets. Low fiber diets are linked to a rise in bowel cancer, heart disease, and blood sugars. It should not be surprising to know that high fiber diets reduce the prevalence of these conditions.

Juice has little to no fiber, whereas apples contain two to four grams. Raspberries, by comparison, have about eight grams per cup. Women require twenty to twenty-five grams of fiber a day, and men need thirty to forty grams per day, but today, adults only ingest about fifteen grams of fiber per day. And unfortunately, children consume even less than in past decades while consuming more salt, sugar, and fat.

You may not have to give up your health or convenience, though. Bring back barley, chickpeas, edamame beans, and chia seeds. Use pressure cookers and/or slow cookers for convenience. Add vegetables, black beans, salsa, and avocado to rice bowls, baked potatoes, or quinoa. Try wrap bread spread with hummus, loaded with vegetables and sprouts, and snacks such as roasted chickpeas or high fiber crackers with bruschetta. At restaurants, try the compromises below for more fiber and proper calories, fat, sugar, and salt.

Eating Out Compromises:

Coffee 2 sugar 2 cream: ~200 cals **or** Milk = 20-30 cals
Egg Muffin with Sausage ~450 cals **or** without Sausage = 300 cals
Large Burger, Large Fries/Soda ~1700 cals **or** Small Burger/Fries/Soda, Fruit ~800 cals

Dinner

10 oz Steak + Caesar Salad + Baked Potato + Butter/Sour Cream ~ >1000 cals.
5 oz Steak + Vegetables + 1 Small Plain Baked Potato + 5oz Wine =

~500 cals

4 oz Steak + Vegetables + Baked Potato/Butter/Sour Cream + Sparkling Water = 500 cals

Totals: ~2500 cals, 2500 milligrams Sodium, 10 g Fiber, minimal vitamins/minerals

or

Total: ~1650 cals; 1500 milligrams Sodium, 17-20 g Fiber, higher vitamins

DOMINO DIET MOMENTS

Busy Thoughts⇒Fight-Flight⇒Malabsorption⇒Risk of Deficiency ⇒ Disease

Calm Thoughts⇒R&R⇒Better Absorption⇒Nourished⇒Healthy Harmony

REFLECTIONS

1. Are you at risk of being overnourished with some foods and undernourished with others? Where do you tend to fall short? Fiber? Omegas?

   _____
   _____
   _____
   _____

2. What adjustment can you make to optimize your cell renewal over the next 120 days?

_____

_____

_____

_____

ACTION STEP

Prescription: Walk twenty to thirty minutes a day or more. Consume three meals and two or three snacks loaded with micronutrients. Practice breathing with R&R. Sleep six to eight hours.

Follow this for one week. If you feel better, continue, and refill this prescription regularly.

SUMMARY

Our diets are becoming deficient in fiber and many other micronutrients, despite the food available to us today, while disease and epidemics are climbing. Is there a correlation? Convenience is important, but health risks are more important. Supplements can be beneficial in some circumstances but detrimental in others. Become wiser, more educated, and empowered by increasing your awareness of preventative health, and in turn, help stop the rise and spread of diseases. Healing is needed now more than ever. Physicians have less time allotted to see you as they try to keep up with the rise in demand. The revolving door of disease management in many cases could be helped with portion control, lifestyle management, and a few old remedies passed on by grandparents from God's pantry to you!

> "The doctor of the future will no longer treat the human frame with drugs, but rather will cure and prevent disease with nutrition."
>
> — Thomas Edison

Tip: Start grocery shopping at the fruit/vegetable aisle. If you wait until the end, you might feel rushed and buy less. Purchase peak season produce for fresh, optimal nutrition and lower prices. Enjoy a variety of superfoods like pomegranate, berries, kiwi, beets, and kale, which have a wide spectrum of nutrients.

AFFIRMATION

Every day I am new; I release old cells. I am renewed with more health. I am health!

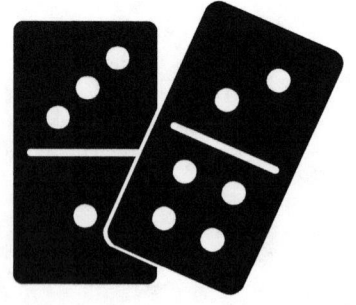

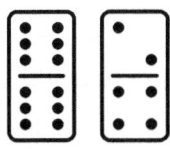

CHAPTER 18

STAYING RESILIENT

"Go the extra mile; it's less crowded there."

— Wayne Dyer

Jody wanted children desperately. After trying for five years, she and her husband decided to try with *in vitro fertilization* (IVF). After a myriad of tests, Jody was diagnosed with *polycystic ovarian syndrome* (PCOS) as the cause of her infertility. She was already stressed, fearing she would not be able to conceive, and then the burden was laid on her shoulders. Her marriage was already strained. Jody had not considered how her sedentary lifestyle and skipping meals were possible contributors to her hormone fluctuations. However, when she saw a dietitian at the direction of her doctor, the benefits of balanced eating were explained. It was then she realized there was still hope and time to take matters into her own hands. Jody's motivation was dialed up by her desire to have children, so she went from lounging to being a "willing walker."

Have you ever felt like everyone is getting away with a frivolous lifestyle, but somehow, you have to follow the straight road to get what you want? Do you feel you need to work harder than others? Although it may now seem like your greatest challenge, it often turns out to be a blessing in disguise.

As you venture into Jody's story, keep the following quote by Thomas Troward in mind. Motivational speaker Bob Proctor placed it in my heart and mind, and I would like to do the same for you.

> My mind is a center of Divine operation. The Divine operation is always for expansion and fuller expression and this means the production of something beyond what has gone before, something entirely new, not included in past experience, though proceeding out of it by an orderly sequence of growth. Therefore, since the Divine cannot change its inherent nature, it must operate in the same manner in me; consequently, in my special world, of which I am the center, it will move forward to produce new conditions, always in advance of any that have gone before.

When Jody received her wakeup call, she realized she needed some new routines. She had never joined a gym or worked with a dietitian before, but her desire propelled her. Although she started slowly at first, with a dietitian and her new gym friend Amber's support, she tried something even newer—she went from a "willing walker" to a "renewed runner." As in the quote above, under her new conditions, her relationship with food became more about eating to fuel her workouts and she stopped eating chips at night. Soon, Amber asked Jody to train with her for a full marathon, all 26.2 miles, in their hometown of Philadelphia. In accepting Amber's invitation, Jody took her goals from "ordinary to extraordinary" and from an orderly sequence of growth.

Whether or not you plan to run a marathon, the quote above is relevant and analogous to a marathon. In a marathon, it is tempting to start the race like a lightning bolt, but in doing so, you risk fizzling out before the end. To break free from your comfort zone as Jody did requires pacing. She needed a "Steady Eddie" approach, with building momentum.

Most marathoners say they tend to hit the wall at about the eighteen-mile mark, where endurance is put to the test. In most cases, when stress hits, we gravitate toward familiar comforts, convincing ourselves nothing is worth the struggle. However, if we stay the course in spite of the challenge, something good begins to happen. Suddenly, a new rhythm kicks in, giving us our second wind. We find ourselves digging in and pulling that little extra from our depths, breaking through the barrier and carrying us the extra miles. The blessings and an orderly sequence of growth are just around the corner. Those blessings also come with a heightened sense of pride because it isn't easy. Can pride exist without a challenge?

Maybe you are at the eighteen-mile mark as you start the eighteenth chapter of this book? Is it time to try something entirely new? Is it time to go from ordinary to extraordinary?

ORDINARY TO EXTRAORDINARY: TOP TEN TIPS

1. Be mindful of your mind, body, spirit (meditate, breathe, pause).
2. Be a beauty sleeper.
3. Build an active lifestyle.
4. Hydrate to concentrate.
5. Break-the-fast with breakfast.
6. Fuel through your day.
7. Eat more whole foods.

8. Refrain from refined (less processed foods, sugar, salt).
9. Use omegas and healthy fats (olive oil, avocado, nuts/nut oils).
10. Replace empty calories with micronutrient-packed meals and snacks.

MINDSHIFT

> "God doesn't call the qualified; God qualifies the called."
>
> — 1 Corinthians 1:27-29

Jody not only made lifestyle changes in health and fitness—on the advice of her dietitian, she began to keep a journal. She was able to pinpoint her stress in connection with her food relationships. Stress was ruling her life from her health to her marriage. The pivotal moment came when she watched a motivational video called *The Mindshift*, narrated by Les Brown. What caught Jody's attention was Brown's description of people changing careers, houses, or spouses as an outward manifestation of the need for inner change. What struck Jody most was when Brown said, "Unless you change inwardly, there's no real change at all."

Jody made her own *mind shift* when she took matters into her own hands and shifted from victim to victor-in-the-making thinking. All the time she had spent assuming everyone had it easier than she did was because they were able to conceive and carry their babies to term. But that didn't mean they weren't struggling elsewhere. Everyone struggles, but those who exemplify resilience are rewarded. This awareness helped Jody drop her victim thinking and take responsibility, which opened doors to friendships, support, and training for a marathon—which was far beyond her perceived abilities from where she once sat.

Jody discovered something else too. She was envious of her new friend Amber because she had a child. But Jody did not know Amber had lost her four-year-old daughter's twin two years earlier. With renewed compassion and understanding, Jody began to release her feeling of being the victim and start managing her stress. She shifted her mind toward gratitude. The inward shift allowed her to support Amber and create a fundraiser in memory of her daughter. She realized, too, that perception played a huge role. After all, which is worse, the pining to have a child or pining from the one you lost?

HEALING WITH HEELS

> "Like my body, I may not control the expiration date, but I certainly influence the quality of the shelf life."
>
> — Gay Hendricks

I realize the concept of your thoughts creating your results can be hard to imagine, in-particular with a diagnosis and especially if you were born with a condition, lived through trauma, or were in an accident you didn't cause. There can be a tendency to feel defensive to this concept or in disbelief. First, you did nothing wrong. Secondly, it wasn't likely conscious, and thirdly, there is no pointing finger since we have all been there. "Everything happens for a reason," is either true or complete bull. Once you do embrace it as truth, you begin to see you do have dominion over your mind, which is where true healing begins.

Jennifer Jiménez, founder of the health and well-being division of the Brave Thinking Institute, states, "When faced with any challenge, first neutralize it from being big to small in your mind. The power breathing you is bigger than your circumstance and provides divine wisdom that leads you to your spiritual growth and Meta-morph-osis!" You make the decisions for your body, not the other way around. What matters is where you place your attention with intention. You choose to stay if you focus on being a victim or you can step out of the conflict. As author and speaker Wayne Dyer said, "Conflict cannot survive without your participation." This includes inner conflict—perhaps even more so. Your decision to participate in conflict is yours alone, just like your inner battle over being active or not.

When you blame your body for not liking exercise, for example, it leaves you wide open for mental conflict and blowing your workout due to TnT (Time and Tiredness). Energy breeds energy, which also means tiredness breeds more tiredness. In reality, going for a walk will likely help you feel more energized. Walking increases healing hormones and helps circulate oxygen-rich blood—both are priceless energizers. Vanity and vitality (V&V) can replace TnT in a heartbeat—and help you sleep better too. More sleep means more serotonin and melatonin; more energy breeds more energy!

You have 1,440 minutes in every day. Imagine or draw two clock faces with numbers marked *a.m.* and *p.m.* Draw lines from one number to the next, indicating the hours you sleep, time spent getting ready for work, driving, working, mealtimes, and how you spend evenings. Distinguish between the hours you spend sitting and moving. How are you spending your time? What adjustments can you make? Recent studies suggest sitting is the new smoking, and many sit ten to twelve hours a day. Where will disease rates go next? This isn't intended as a guilt trip but rather an assessment of the other T in TnT—time. Identifying how you spend your time can help you set better, more realistic goals. Jody went from victim thinking to running marathons. Although she could only run for one minute at first, she took that step. I asked avid hiker Rob Burris how he climbed some of the highest mountains in the world. "I did it with the mantra 'step, step, repeat.'"

The good news is you do not have to join a gym or run a marathon. Puttering around the house works too. Walking thirty minutes all at once or in ten-minute intervals throughout the day adds up, and either one is effective in lowering the risk of disease. Pedometers can help measure your activity and allow you to set goals accordingly. The average office worker takes 4,000 steps a day, while the goal for optimal benefit is 10,000 steps a day. To release weight, you will need an average of 12,000 steps a day, along with a balanced diet. If you spend ten minutes doing other activities like biking, it equates to about 1,000 steps. For a holistic lifestyle, many national guidelines suggest moderate physical activity for 150 minutes a week, two days should include strength training, and one or two days should include flexibility exercises such as yoga.

Treadmills and gyms are great, but neither existed once upon a time. They are not necessary. Start with a priceless walk. Don't wait for a perfect routine—construct one in your mind while you walk. Waiting for a perfect plan is really just procrastination. Get creative and power-up with ten-minute power moves. Wash walls one day, floors the next. Get the kids involved. Lethargy can turn into low-self-esteem, but movement can generate confidence. Even water goes stagnant sitting too long. You are designed to move, and the benefits are more than worth the effort.

YOUR TRUE BENEFITS

> "Walking is man's best medicine."
>
> — Hippocrates

It seems responsible, staying at a job you no longer love for the health benefits; it's true that illness comes with a price. However, stresses at work can create illness, while anticipating illness can draw it to you. It seems counterintuitive, does it not? Why does society place more emphasis on employee benefits and assuming illness instead of the *healthy benefits* of promoting a healthier lifestyle? While not true for everyone, it does appear many people pay more for their vehicle's maintenance than their own. Fortunately, you are farther ahead, so you can also help others understand the health benefits of exercise.

How Exercise Reduces Common Diseases

Heart Disease: increases good cholesterol and lowers bad cholesterol.

Blood Sugars: improves insulin resistance and weight management.

High Blood Pressure: improves circulation and weight management.

Osteoporosis: builds bone density and muscle for added agility and protection against fractures.

Digestive Disorders: improves circulation to stomach nerves.

Most Cancers: decreases inflammation, improves immune system, cellular communication.

Mental Health: increases serotonin, vitality, and self-esteem.

Obesity: weight management, increased serotonin, more energy.

Sleep Hygiene: boosts serotonin and melatonin, leads to better appetite control.

Immune System Health: improves hormones and cell communication.

Arthritis: improves circulation, reduces inflammation, and aids overall vascular health.

Hormone Balance: allows enhancement of the parasympathetic system.

Thyroid Diseases: assist in offsetting added weight and increasing metabolism.

WEATHERING "STORMS" WITH SUPPORT

> "Fall seven times; stand up eight."
>
> — Japanese Proverb

A friend of mine lived on acreage in the country surrounded by trees, except for one exposed, barren area. He had an abundant supply of trees in a marshy, well-protected area of his property and decided to transplant a few to liven up the exposed area. He transplanted the trees from protected, marshy soil to barren, exposed, sandy soil. The trees were uprooted and immersed into a whole new ecosystem. They became vulnerable and dependent on ropes for support, tender loving care, and fertilizer for nutrients. Tending to them was like tending to Goldilocks—they needed water but not too much or it might erode the sand, not too little or they might wither. The ropes were not too tight to allow enough bend, but not too loose to risk the trees falling over.

You might be adjusting to a new ecosystem too. You might need TLC and support too. Are you surrounded by those who support you, or by people who restrict you and grip you too tightly? How do you provide support? While you may not be able to leave one ecosystem for another, be mindful of your surroundings and find a "partner in believing." Jody and Amber crossed the finish line, not only completing their marathon but going on to Rome the following March to complete another! In marching forth, Jody expected a little more weight release, but the unexpected happened. She noted a few missed cycles and it wasn't PCOS. Jody was pregnant.

> "Be like a tree. Stay grounded, connect with your roots. Turn over a new leaf. Bend before you break. Enjoy your unique natural beauty. Keep growing."
>
> — Joanne Rapies

DOMINO DIET MOMENT

Victim Thoughts⇒Fight-Flight⇒Anxious/Tired/Illness Focused⇒More tired⇒Disease

Victory Thoughts⇒R&R⇒Vitality⇒Active Life⇒More Vitality⇒Health Harmony

REFLECTIONS

1. What is calling you to march forth? Is it a marathon or a 5K race perhaps?

   _____
   _____
   _____
   _____

2. Who is supporting you or holding you back? Which person are you?

   _____
   _____
   _____
   _____

ACTION STEP

Using the breathing technique discussed earlier, tap into your creative side aligning with your R&R and recall something you are grateful for. Ask what step you can take to go from ordinary to extraordinary. Is finding a "partner in believing" a step for you?

SUMMARY

You have a reason for being here. You have pushed through the eighteen-mile mark, despite your circumstances. You are making a "mindshift" and changing inwardly while transplanting yourself into a new way of life, one step at a time. You are becoming more resilient and discovering your true, authentic self. You are in a special world that you are the center of. Something is calling you to march forth in an orderly sequence of growth that you are being qualified for. With "heels to heal," ready for the long run, add a little TLC from a partner who believes in you to your true health benefits.

AFFIRMATION

"An obstacle is often a stepping stone."

— Prescott Hippocrates

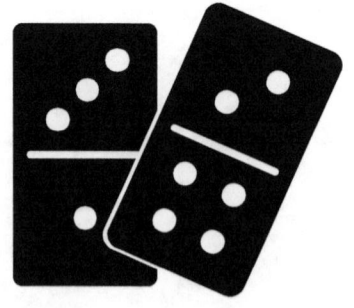

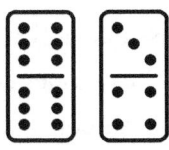

CHAPTER 19

CALENDARIZING

"To accomplish great things, we must not only act but also dream, not only plan but also believe."

— Anatole France

As you know, waiting for the perfect time to take steps toward optimal health is procrastination. Planning and waiting for Monday, the following Monday, the new year, or the following new year is just a delaying tactic. Time will keep passing by unless you develop tools and strategies now.

I remember the first time I heard a motivational speaker. It wasn't my first experience listening to speakers and professors, but I had previously found them dull. Elizabeth Jeffries, author of *The Heart of Leadership*, was different. She walked on stage beaming in her coat of many colors, red shoes, and a remote in hand—the clicker was for the all-new flashy PowerPoint slides. Slide one appeared and said in bold letters "Housekeeping." Thankfully, she quickly moved on to the next few slides. Then she said, "You will never know your career mission until you are on your personal mission, as the two are inextricably linked." My eyes grew wide, and my heart opened even wider. It felt like she reached through the crowded audience to tap my shoulder. It wasn't just a lecture in science or biology—except for how she spoke to my beaming heart. I was working on a Bachelor of Science degree, but she inspired me to become a motivational speaker too. I was awestruck by 80 percent of what she said. What would have happened if she had droned on about housekeeping instead? I would not have found the path she laid before me.

How would you measure the content of your time? Is housekeeping or social media distracting you 80 percent of the time, leaving 20 percent for things that truly fulfill you?

The truth of the matter is that *delay, distraction, and dissuasion* are indicators that you may need a tool and/or a structure of support, and your calendar is a step in that direction. Your calendar can help schedule 20 percent of your time for housekeeping, like dust Mondays, windows Tuesdays, floor Wednesdays, and so on. The only thing that really needs dusting off is your precious dream. Place more of what you love on your calendar so 80 percent of your time is spent there. You have ideas, dreams, and more. Think of a water truck coming to your home to fill your new backyard pool. Are preparations and supports ready for the water? The ideas and dreams will be lost with nothing to gather them.

> "Time is free, but it is priceless; you cannot own it, but you can use it. You can't keep it, but you can spend it; once you've used it, you can never get it back."
>
> — Harvey Mackay

ASSESS, ADAPT, CORRECT

> "By thought, the thing you want is brought to you; by action you receive it."
>
> — Wallace Wattles

Are you a perfectionist? It could be holding you back. It sets up all-or-nothing thinking, another form of delay that keeps you from experimenting. If you see your steps as a trial and error experiment, you can adjust as you go along. Now that you have your calendar with the 80:20 rule as your template, you can absolutely create a life you love. Your calendar creates a productivity rhythm with permission for rest and recovery (the other R&R). Take an honest look at ways to stay the course and avoid burnout too. Sometimes you need to adjust, adapt, correct, and even release things that no longer serve you.

Make a list of what you *need* and *want* to accomplish. Then, using your calendar, begin shifting your time allowing what you *want* to be front and center. In this assessment, you have options to: 1) Continue, 2) Limit, 3) Omit, 4) Delegate, and 5) (identify to-dos to) Begin. You will have an opportunity to explore this list at the end of the chapter also, but for now, think about what you *want*, like dance classes or meditating. Would limiting social media time or hiring someone to manage your social media be beneficial? Can you delegate more to staff or family? With experimenting, you can always adjust and adapt. Michelangelo was once asked how he managed to sculpt his masterpiece *David*. He said, "You chip away the stone that does not look like David." What can you chip away that does not look like your dream?

POOR MONDAYS

"Create a life you love, one you don't need a vacation from."

— Unknown

Do you find the days of the week have a certain energy? You look forward to Fridays, dread Mondays, enjoy Saturdays and Sundays with family, but Mondays are back to work with rules and diets. Poor Mondays. No wonder they're dreaded—up until now, that is. What if each day contained something you love, including Monday?

You have explored your dream-vision and are taking steps toward it. You are aware paradigms may try to hold you back. With your 80:20 rule on your calendar, you can veer away from distraction and dissuasion. However, are you wondering, "How can I fill my schedule with what I love when it is packed with what I don't?" Look a month ahead, and place a few steps or goals you can take and place on your calendar before the time is spoken for with things not in the land of your dreams. If you shovel the piles while they are small, you can start even today. Many of the brilliant authors and philosophers quoted earlier in this book suggest making five- to ten-minute power moves, as something is better than nothing. You know the saying, "If you want something done, ask someone who is busy to do it." Get busy with your own to-do first. Start small by walking after work and having the kids take over preparations for Taco Tuesday (refer to my website www.TheDomino-Diet.com for *Kids Can Cook* recipes). Perhaps your child will discover a hidden chef within. If you feel uneasy about letting go, explore your hidden fears and try to take control of them. Is perfectionism loitering there? Take imperfect action on behalf of what you love. Allow your schedule to serve you. The goal is to omit the words, "I am too busy," also known as procrastination. When you do, you will soon embrace every day, including Mondays.

WISHING OR KISSING

> "You are never given a wish without also being given the power to make it come true."
>
> — Richard Bach

Studies show that 70 percent of people wish for a better life, but believe it is possible for others but not themselves. The truth is few plan and even fewer take steps. You can read all the books and take all the courses, but they remain mere entertainment unless you implement them. "Visioning" is a verb involving action with images held in your mind. To bring them into fruition, they require your physical action steps to complete the circuit, and in doing so, you are also telling your subconscious, "I'm saying yes to my dream."

If your past efforts to release weight resulted in a five-pound decrease each year for five years, where would you be today? Does it seem manageable or daunting? Don't take on more than you can handle. Deciding to join a gym and go five days a week for two hours each time is a challenge and can cause you to give up. Was it the gym or the goal? Too many goals at once tend to fail. If you set ten goals, chances are you will achieve one or none of them. When you set four to ten goals, you might achieve one or two, but if you have two or three goals, odds are you will achieve two or three of them. Your subconscious prefers smaller experiments overall. For example, incorporating one fruit or vegetable at meals for one week has staying power.

Remember Pamela, who enjoyed golfing with her mother? She started slowly, golfing one evening a week. Her enjoyment and success allowed her to stay the course, and soon she was golfing three nights a week as her confidence grew—allowing the unexpected to happen. Her teammate Erin mentioned she was taking online courses in pursuit of a master's degree. It inspired Pamela to finish her education degree. With a scheduled plan that included more time for activities, Pamela released twenty pounds and gained a new career. With baby steps, she went from wishing to success by keeping it simple.

HAPPY NEW YEAR

> "No one can go back in time to change what has happened. So, work on your present to make yourself a wonderful future."
>
> — Unknown

Is there any other time of the year that rings in the word diets like New Year's Eve? Personally, I enjoy setting resolutions and writing bucket lists. I know not everyone shares this view. If, however, you had success with resolutions, chances are you would welcome them each and every year. Sadly, they are a double-edged sword that cuts both ways unless you know how to sharpen your skills.

The bad cut:

1. Waiting for New Year's can be worse than waiting for Mondays to change as a delay tactic. In the end, it means you may not be ready just because it's a new year.
2. If the bar is set too high, goals are less achievable and become discouraging.
3. The swings in extremes from Christmas indulgences to restrictive eating can alarm your subconscious, causing it to panic.
4. Goals are set in the vibration of guilt.

The good cut:

1. A collective consciousness is happening at the same time around New Year's, making it easier to find a partner in believing.
2. Setting goals means one might stick.
3. You might find seasonal deals on gym memberships or equipment.
4. Your calendar is new, like a clean slate.

If you fall, get back up and create a new fresh start, setting another New Year's Day within the same calendar year. Although January 1 marks the new year in North America, many other cultures start their new year on a different date. Every day can be the start of a new year. If you take one step a month, you will take twelve steps ahead, or you can wait 120 days and start the year with a brand-new you with your new red blood cells every 120 days too.

IT'S A BRAND-NEW DAY

> "You can't wait for all the lights to turn green before heading out of town."
>
> — Zig Ziglar

You have access to tools: your calendar, goals, dreams/vision, and the top ten tips in the previous chapter. Maybe you have 120 days already in the making and/or twelve months scheduled on the calendar. Many people struggle to pull all the pieces together to create and implement a daily system. Below are examples you can customize for your days.

The Early Bird

6:00-6:15	wake—meditate/generate gratitude
6:15-7:15	shower and get ready—set intentions, affirmations, read vision while getting ready
7:15-7:30	breakfast
7:30-8:00	to work—motivational podcast
8:00-12:00	work
12:00-1:00	pause three minutes, eat lunch, walk for fifteen to twenty minutes
1:00-5:00	work
5:00-5:30	drive home—favorite tunes
5:30-6:30	pause three minutes—supper/prepare night snack and next-day meals
6:30-7:00	active/walk/kids
7:00-8:00	favorite hobby
8:00-9:00	downtime—health snack
9:00-10:30	bed—read/reflect/journal/set intentions/affirmation

Midnight Owl

7:00-7:45	awake—shower/gratitude/affirmations/intentions/read vision
7:45-8:00	to work—motivational podcast
8:00-12:00	pause breakfast/meditate five minutes before work
12:00-1:00	pause three minutes, eat lunch, walk fifteen to thirty minutes
1:00-5:00	work
5:00-5:30	home—favorite tunes
5:30-6:30	pause/supper/prep tomorrow's meals
6:30-8:00	active time—walk/kids
8:00-9:00	favorite hobby, snack
9:00-11:00	downtime
11:00-12:00	meditate/read/set intention/affirmation

> "Goals are good for setting a direction, but systems are best for making progress. A handful of problems arise when you spend too much time thinking about your goals and not enough time designing your systems."
>
> — James Clear

APP FOR THAT

There are many tools to help you monitor and stay on track with your calendar and goals: phone notifications, calendars, electronic reminders, smart home gadgets, etc. You can also use these to set reminders along the way to help keep you motivated, including the use of positive affirmations. Try sending an email to yourself using the "delayed delivery" option for future dates or extra tempting days like Easter when extra chocolate is around with notes of inspiration. Don't forget to reward yourself with items like new runners, outfits, or cologne. Recognize those times you put the doughnut down and walked away and toss a coin in a jar to mark your success. It all adds up. Plus, there are plenty of apps to help track your lifestyle changes that go well beyond weight alone. Measure your energy levels, productivity, and your dream. You can even create vision boards to use as your phone background. Also, look at your calendar, noting the celebrations ahead, including birthdays, anniversaries, etc. There are at least twelve special occasions and fifty-two Fridays/weekends, so approximately 100 days out of 365 days of temptations per the dates below. Use the 80/20 rule to plan and enjoy your special occasions while using the majority to work toward your dreams.

January New Year's Day
February Valentine's Day
March St. Patrick's Day
April Easter/Passover
May Mother's Day
June Father's Day
July Fourth of July
August Summer Vacation
September Labor Day
October Halloween
November Thanksgiving
December Christmas/Hanukkah/Kwanzaa

From the start of the year in January for most to the end of the year with Christmas, there are special occasions generally each month. With the added birthdays and anniversaries, weekends and vacations away, they add up. Be realistic and plan to enjoy these by marking them on the calendar too. No guilt—just enjoy, but with the intention that you plan to get back on track again. Avoid the "All or Nothing Thinking" and adopt the 80/20 rule!

TURNING A YEAR AROUND

> "Strength doesn't come from what you can do. It comes from overcoming the things you once thought you couldn't."
>
> — Rikki Rogers

It was the start of a new year and Steve's dream was slowly emerging. His headaches from drowning his feelings in a bottle and the painful gout in his toes created a mindshift. He heard a whisper telling him to start playing guitar. However, his schedule was "too full." His all-or-nothing thinking required a change in perspective.

Time to practice never made Steve's calendar. It didn't seem worthwhile unless he could free up a full hour in the evening. Even when he found the time, practice was often forgotten. One evening, while in a mood, he walked past his guitar en route to splitting wood outside (delay and distract). He placed a log in the splitter, and while his mind drifted to angry thoughts, he cut off his right index finger. He rushed to the hospital with his finger in a bag of ice. The surgeon was able to reattach the finger, but told Steve he might never have feeling in it again.

You know the saying, "You never really appreciate something until you lose it"? Well, losing something can change your perception too. Steve's experience changed him completely. He suddenly felt empowered and compelled to do whatever it took to regain the ability to play guitar. After the surgery, just plying for fifteen minutes was noteworthy and acted as his dangling carrot. He changed his lifestyle to include healthy eating, supplements, and exercise. Dexterity returned after diligently adhering to his physiotherapy schedule and arming his body with micronutrients. In fact, his surgeon had never seen such a significant injury heal so fast. Although Steve spent a few years in his victim story, it all turned around when he latched onto his dream and turned it into a hero's journey. Steve added guitar practice to his calendar wherever he had a fifteen-minute opening and it all turned around—he had no idea what he was really in for.

DOMINO DIET MOMENTS

Christmas Indulge⇒Panic⇒Guilt⇒Unrealistic Goals⇒Same Challenge Every Year

Christmas Eve/Day⇒Love⇒Guilt-Free⇒Walks⇒Realistic Goals⇒Every Year Better

REFLECTIONS

1. Assess how you spend your twenty-four hours. Make a list of what you would like to…

    Omit
    Start
    Limit
    Delegate
    Keep

2. What schedule would you create for your optimal brand-new day?

   _____
   _____
   _____
   _____

ACTION STEP

Search the available apps to schedule, monitor, and track your goals. Try a yearly-view wall calendar and schedule a rhythm of productivity, recovery, special days, and rest. Use the 80/20 rule, notifications, and pop-up reminders for rewards too.

SUMMARY

You cannot change without changing your mind. Bringing what you love to the front of your mind as part of a theme on your calendar creates a new life for you. Use your calendar as an extension of yourself and as a support structure filled with love and what will serve you. Start on any day, including New Year's Day. Baby steps will help you climb and stay on track. Imagine a year filled with what you love. If you fall off course, correct and reassess. What needs to be omitted, delegated, limited, kept, or started? It's not all or nothing. It's not about Christmas. It's about Christmas being a month long, camping being a season long, and Fridays for a lifetime. Happy New Year and Happy Brand-New Day! You can go from wishing to kissing!

> "You don't create a great life; you create great moments that lead you to a great life."
>
> — Mary Morrissey

AFFIRMATION

I am beautiful. I see the beauty in every day!

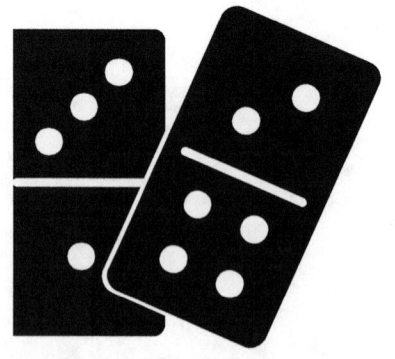

SECTION 7

THE SIXTH DOMINO— EMBRACING YOUR RESULTS

DOMINO DIET FORMULA:

Thoughts⇒Breath⇒Hormones⇒Feelings⇒Actions⇒ **Results**⇒…Freedom

---

"Since life is *infinite*, the concept of an ultimate destiny is inconceivable. When we understand that consciousness is the only reality, we know that it is the only creator. This means that your consciousness is the creator of your destiny."

— Neville

By now, you are seeing results using the tools we've discussed thus far to design a life you will love, and you are no longer living by default. You have begun noticing your thoughts, which leads to paying attention to your breathing and the connection both have to your body chemistry. You are releasing and renewing from the inside out, down to the cellular level. Now that you are seeing results, how do you stay the course? How many stories have you heard about recurring illnesses or losing weight only to find it again? You may feel you can release weight, but you gain it back again. Is this because maintenance is misunderstood? Is there a common denominator in honeymoons that leads to divorce, in bankruptcies after lotto wins, or in weight gains after a quick fix diet? Why do some sustain their results while others do not?

We'll explore those questions in this final section.

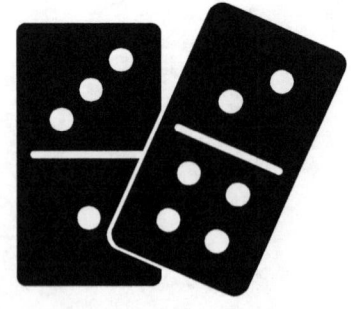

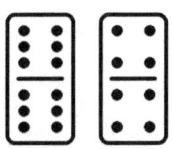

CHAPTER 20

LOST AND FOUND WEIGHT

"When I lost all of my excuses, I found my results."

—Unknown

In 1979, my parents took my brother, sister, and me on an Adventure Land getaway. After a few rounds on the rollercoasters and Ferris wheels, hunger led us to the Wonderland Cafe. Each of us grabbed our own tray and slid it along a metal conveyer. Our parents said we could choose whatever we wanted! Hardly able to see over the railing, we proudly made our selections. With trays full, we eagerly waited for Mom to pay. As she reached for her purse, her eyes suddenly widened, and she let out a loud gasp. With trembling hands, she recalled earlier setting down her purse and mistakenly leaving it. Then, like a movie scene playing in reverse, we moved backward, putting each item back from where it came from and the empty trays back on the rack.

Back then, cash and traveler's checks were the norm. Mom had a purse, and so by default, she was elected to carry everything—passports and all. Hunger was one thing. The real panic came when we had to figure out how to get home. To our relief, a good Samaritan returned the purse to the lost and found!

Do you know the feeling of losing something? It becomes etched in your mind, especially when you have an emotional attachment to the thing you lost. Your subconscious sears the experience into your mind. Same goes for the relief when you find a lost item.

The desire to lose weight is so prevalent you might have been tempted to jump to this chapter first rather than sift through the pages of this book. Of course, rushing to the symptom level (weight gain) for an answer isn't what is new and precisely what may be backward. Buying a fast pass to weight loss seems worthwhile at first, but you risk going up and down and back around like a roller coaster. Having read this book from the beginning, though, you know the word *loss* has a negative undertone. Could it trigger your subconscious to find it (whatever it may be) again?

What if the word *loss* was replaced with *release*? You release carbon dioxide through your respiratory system, where fat is oxidized, and your subconscious doesn't try to find your CO_2 again. Envisioning weight release while walking can be quite empowering while releasing cortisol too. The idea of release is something your body is accustomed to. From this mindset, you will *find* vital health holistically, connecting all areas in your life for sustained results.

> "How you do one thing is how you do everything."
>
> — Mary Morrissey

MAINTENANCE MINDSET: A "WEALTH OF HEALTH"

"There's birth, there's death, and in between there's maintenance."

— Tom Robbins

You know the saying, born with a silver spoon in their mouth, meaning born into wealth. Perhaps this statement would be best followed by a disclaimer that being born into wealth doesn't guarantee sustained wealth.

What would you do if you won a million dollars? Pay off your home? Buy a sports car? Save it? If you spend $200,000, leaving $800,000, are you still a millionaire? If you spend $20,000 on a trip, you are a $980,000 heir, but no longer a millionaire.

When Rob and his wife Susan checked their weekly lotto ticket, their life changed overnight—$1.2 million worth of change. A financial adviser suggested investing their windfall. However, the opportunity to move closer to Susan's family, to be near her father who had fallen ill, took precedence. Happily, they moved to a new home near her parents and helped them renovate their home. The $1.2 million became $400,000. Maintaining their new home now meant finding work. Even modest living comes with money fluctuations.

You've heard it before—the majority of lotto winners end up broke. Sustained results require a maintenance mindset, and maintenance itself requires renovating too.

As stated earlier, everything is energy, and it's dynamic, never static. Even a bear in hibernation and dormant trees are in a state of flux.

Nothing is truly solid or paused. Despite the naked eye's point of view, everything, right down to the book you are holding, contains vibrating particles. Your fit friend doesn't stay fit without maintaining fitness. Maintaining is a verb, therefore, an action. The grass is greener on the other side because someone is maintaining it. Millionaires stay millionaires by managing (maintaining) their money. When it comes to weight release or health, though, maintenance is often misunderstood. Achieving an ideal weight or cholesterol level isn't just a destination. Once you arrive, your actions keep you there. Like the farmer who plants a crop, there is more work upfront, removing rocks and roots and preparing the field, but once the crop is planted, the work doesn't stop.

Unfortunately, quick fix diets do not prepare you to maintain your new physique once you've achieved it. You will burn fewer calories without the added weight unless you build enough muscle too. You need a custom program that considers everything—age, hormones, muscle growth, cell repair, injuries, illness, and activity. When it comes to maintaining your wealth of health, make sure it comes with a prescription specific to you and a healthy maintenance mindset.

PRESCRIPTION TO MAINTAINING HEALTH

"It is not the thing believed in that brings an answer to man's prayers; the answer to prayer results when the individual's subconscious mind responds to the mental picture or thought in his mind."

— Joseph Murphy

Chronic disease management often requires specific medications and/or lifestyle modifications. Some people require medications just to stay alive. Despite the positive effects of medications, there can be negative ones, too. Below are common chronic diseases, each with their specific treatments. What they have in common, though, is how they are better managed with a healthy lifestyle. In fact, those diseases such as high blood pressure, cholesterol, diabetes, etc. that may require medications can improve when combining lifestyle changes, to the point of lowering dosage requirements and their coinciding side effects. In some cases, medications are discontinued altogether!

COMMON CHRONIC DISEASES

Arthritis: There are varying types of arthritis and, therefore, various remedies. For osteoarthritis, Vitamin D and calcium are often suggested. A diet rich in omegas, essential fatty acids, and/or supplements can be beneficial as well as limiting salt, alcohol, and caffeine. Activity, even in small intervals, can improve circulation, reduce inflammation, balance hormones, and manage pain. Some individuals report having pain relief from taking the herb white willow bark available in herb tea or capsule form.

Blood Pressure: Often, high pressure occurs due to blockages in circulation from plaque buildup and/or a thicker volume of blood. Limiting salt to less than 1500-2000 milligrams a day can help blood volume. Walking is good for circulation, weight management, increasing good cholesterol (HDL), lowering bad cholesterol (LDL), and lowering plaque buildup. Also, walking and meditation can help offset the fight-flight stress hormones. Finally, a diet rich in antioxidants, fiber, omegas, and other micronutrients can be beneficial.

Cholesterol: There are medications to help manage heart disease. Cholesterol is produced in your liver as well as consumed in the diet through animal products. Not all fat sources contain cholesterol (plant sources do not) but your total amount of fat intake needs consideration in regards to calories and weight management. Increasing HDL can help offset LDL levels. Think of LDL as balls of cotton that sticks to the walls of your arteries and HDL as marbles that can push the LDL away. With increased activity, fiber, and omegas, HDL are often increased too. Lowering LDL can also occur with consuming less than 300 milligrams of cholesterol per day, and limiting saturated fats (hardened fats like butter, palm oil, and lard) is suggested. Butter only contains eleven milligrams (keeping portions in mind) of cholesterol per teaspoon compared to 200 milligrams in an egg. Therefore, recommendations average around one egg a day if your cholesterol levels are in range and three or four eggs per week if they are high. Egg whites, however, are cholesterol-free. Liver and organ meat are high in cholesterol, while meat contains about 100 milligrams in three ounces (the size of a deck of cards). Aim for healthy fatty acids such as avocado, nuts/nut oils, olive oil, flax, or sesame oils, with portion control and small, frequent meals.

Depression: We are more aware of mental disorders now, so we have more medications available. They can be necessary. Still, lifestyle management, like getting plenty of vitamin D from sun exposure and/or supplements, is also important. Additional lifestyle changes are also helpful, like limiting alcohol (a known depressant), proper sleep hygiene, walking, listening to music, meditation, deep breathing, and a nourishing diet with less caffeine. These can all assist with blood sugar control, anxiety/panic attacks, hormonal balance, and overall stress. Also limiting screen time with negative messages and replacing it with social interactions and support groups is helpful. Finally, St. John's Wort may be a helpful herb for mild depression.

Diabetes: Type 1, Type 2 along with gestational diabetes (in pregnancy) all can be mitigated with lifestyle changes. These forms of diabetes are different with regards to how they arise, but they have common management regimes. They involve blood glucose monitoring and adjustments to sugar consumption. The hormone insulin is needed in Type 1 diabetes for survival, while Type 2 may or may not rely on insulin and/or oral agents. Some studies suggest using cinnamon for blood sugar control in Type 2 diabetes, but this usage has had variable results and dosages vary. As always, weight management, small and frequent meals—especially with portion control (fewer calories, fat, salt, and sugar), activity, and sleep hygiene can lower the risk of complications such as heart disease.

Gout: A painful form of arthritis, also known as the King's Disease, gout is caused by high levels of uric acid creating crystals around joints like in toes. Uric acid is formed by breaking down purines; therefore, a low purine diet (fewer organ meats, red meat, some seafood, asparagus, bone broth, spinach) and limiting alcohol, sugary foods, and caffeine is suggested. Weight reduction and tolerated activity, plus increased water intake, is also highly encouraged. Some have success with a diet high in cherries and/or black cherry juice concentrate. Although many people require medication for gout, these medications have possible side effects, making lifestyle changes the superior choice overall.

Reflux: Between the bottom of the esophagus and top of your stomach is a valve called the cricopharyngeal sphincter. Pressures from spicy foods, tomato, citrus, mint, chocolate, caffeine, fatty foods, alcohol, eating too fast, and/or lying down too soon after meals can cause pressure on the valve to open. Sitting in crouched positions for long periods can create symptoms also. Some may undergo procedures to diagnose what is called a hiatal hernia. When stomach acids rise between the diaphragm and/or chest or throat, heartburn and chest pains can result. Allow more than two hours for digestion before lying down, eat small and frequent meals, and use breath techniques, stress management, activity, and weight control. When chest pain occurs, never assume it's heartburn—visit your closest hospital!

Thyroid: Various thyroid conditions often alter metabolism and weight and cause fatigue, depression, temperature intolerance, and digestive issues. Medications are available, depending on TSH, T4, and T3 (hormone) levels. While there is controversy regarding foods that hinder or improve, an overall healthy lifestyle is encouraged. Also controversial is consuming kelp or high iodine foods, which actually have minimal risk.

Several other diseases and details, especially related to digestive and sleep disorders (i.e., sleep apnea), exist beyond those I have mentioned. The bottom line is that a prescription, including lifestyle strategies, is recommended, and I would be remiss if I didn't highlight these advantages. If lifestyle changes were emphasized and implemented more, perhaps disease rates would go down. This isn't news. However, up until now, implementing a healthy mindset first hasn't been the top priority for many traditional medicines. Putting the *heal* back into health and going beyond just treating symptoms may provide a new way and a new prescription with no negative side effects and unlimited refills.

Prescription: The Domino Diet Formula Rx

Directions: Envision your dream. Develop positive thinking and sleep habits. Use positive affirmations, meditation, and breath techniques for more R&R and hormonal balance. Consume small, frequent meals high in micronutrients and adopt an active lifestyle.

Dosage: Suggest a minimum of once a day and/or more as needed.

Side Effects: May create happiness, peace, and optimal well-being with fulfilled dreams.

Refills: Unlimited and covered by your health benefits provider—your mind.

PRACTICING AND MASTERING

"To become a master at any skill, it takes the total effort of your: heart, mind, and soul working together in tandem."

— Maurice Young

The following strategies with sustained results are practiced by masters:

1. Set realistic goals with vitality over vanity. Be aware that thoughts happen first.
2. Stay active. Eat small, frequent meals. Use food journals.
3. Get support from a *mastermind* group or *mentor*.
4. Follow your *intuition* and take steps.
5. Be mindful with gratitude.
6. Visualize your dream daily with a *be, do, have* vs. *have, be, do* mindset.
7. Be willing to continue growing in the face of discomfort.
8. Get back on track after falling.
9. Know that success in all areas of life is connected.
10. Use a holistic approach and a willingness to be empowered.

MASTERMIND MENTOR

"You are the master of your fate, the captain of your soul."

— Napoleon Hill

I started work at 5:00 a.m. The homemade bread needed to rise and then bake to be ready for the morning customers, timed so they could smell the fresh bread.

There is a science to making bread, every ingredient having a dual function. You need lukewarm water for the yeast to rise and to provide moisture. You use flour to form the dough and the gluten it contains to support the rising process. Sugar has three roles: 1) feed the yeast, 2) add taste, 3) caramelize the sugar for toasty brown bread. Salt adds flavor and stabilizes yeast fermentation to strengthen your dough and prevent holes and funnels.

While there are plenty of recipes for making bread that may seem easy to follow, there are also many variables. Temperature, humidity, and even the type of flour can alter the quality of your bread. My grandmothers were masters who could knead, mix, and adjust for stickiness without overmixing, just by feel. Working with a mentor can help you mold things into shape more efficiently and often quicker than trying on your own. Someone to guide and cheer you on is helpful in most situations. Having someone who has mastered what you are hoping to achieve to support you is priceless.

YOUR INVISIBLE VOICE

> "Have the courage to follow your heart and intuition. They somehow already know what you truly want to become. Everything else is secondary."
>
> — Steve Jobs

You probably have many gifts, but one of the most important is your intuition. We've all felt the gentle nudge or gut feeling when something seems wrong or right despite all logic. Robert Collier, author of the 1925 book *Secret of the Ages*, said, "There constantly resided within you, a mind that is all-wise, all-powerful, a mind that is entirely apart from the mind which you consciously use in your everyday affairs, yet which is one with it."

When you become present, your intuition strengthens in providing guidance. It will increase with your willingness to listen, and you carry it everywhere. As you learn more from your intuition, there will be no need for counting calories; you will eat according to your nutritional needs. The voice will seem familiar but quiet, never booming or nagging, and it always moves in the direction of harmony. Just as you can trust that the invisible electricity in your home will power your lights, you can trust your intuition as your invisible power, and it's free and unlimited! Even more, when you develop it, it moves you in directions you may not have otherwise thought of with your logical mind.

OUT OF THE BLUE

> "If one advances confidently in the direction of his dreams, and endeavors to live the life which he has imagined, he will meet with a success unexpected in common hours. He will put some things behind, will pass an invisible boundary; new, universal, more liberal laws will begin to establish themselves around and within him; or the old laws be expanded and interpreted in his favor in a more liberal sense, and he will live with the license of a higher order of beings."
>
> — Henry David Thoreau

I saved every penny. I was eighteen and making $5 an hour. My friends partied every weekend, but if I joined, my purse strings were tight. My new motto was, "Every $5 here is better spent there." Peer pressure did not sway me, which was unusual. I still craved acceptance. Still, this dream started to change me.

The dream was inspired by a combination of the movie *Crocodile Dundee* and my friend from New Zealand. When my "Kiwi" friend invited me to visit, it ignited a feeling I couldn't let go of. After saving enough money, my boyfriend (who later became my first husband) and I left for the land down under to backpack for a six months!

A few months in, we ventured to Stradbroke Island where I stood on a cliff, taking in the view of the most beautiful aqua-blue water, sweeping onto miles of white sands—a picture-perfect postcard. By evening, though, the winds had picked up and the locals started battening down hatches. Shutter doors were closing, and latches were latching. A cyclone? Hurricane? Typhoon? I had no idea what was coming. All I knew was palm trees were spitting coconuts, debris was flying, and the rain was coming down in sheets. We hunkered down for three whole days waiting for the monsoon to pass.

I wasn't much of a reader, which I attribute to the mandatory books in school, like *1984*, *Zen and the Art of Motorcycle Maintenance*, and Shakespeare that I found boring. During the monsoon, though, with little to do, the book *Dream Catcher* by Monica Hughes caught my eye. Surprisingly, I escaped the storm to a whole other realm. As far as I was concerned, the storm could last until my sabbatical in the mystical world was over. We booked a three-hour scuba diving tour, but like Gilligan, we ended up marooned on a gorgeous island—where I inhaled a book, inspiring the reader, and later the writer, in me.

When the storm finally ceased and the birds chirped again and the water reflected the glowing sun, I eagerly walked to the cliff to take one last look at the magnificent view. This time, though, my heart sank. The ocean had returned to the sparkling blue as though nothing had happened, but the beach was no longer white. The ocean had coughed up miles and miles of rubbish, as the Aussies call it. Tires, bikes, plastic, seaweed, and even a washing machine littered the shoreline. Just days previous, I had resonated with this picture-perfect postcard of a serene beach scene. I felt so saddened. Then I heard a voice say, "See the good." I didn't call it my inner voice or intuition then, but it was the same voice I heard egging me on to go on the trip itself. It said, "The ocean holds no grudge against a storm that cleans." In fact, the ocean didn't just go back to normal—it was even cleaner than before, chaos and all.

I didn't see it at the time, as the quote at the beginning of this chapter suggests. But by taking a step, saving money, and endeavoring despite naysayers, I allowed the Universe to step toward me. Through an invisible boundary, new universal laws organized what would be revealed next.

Standing on a dock in Perth, Australia, while once again staring at the blue ocean, I heard the voice again, "I will be a dietitian." I didn't even know what a dietitian was! I believe the steps leading to the land "down under" gave me a new confidence that allowed more steps to be revealed beyond my logical thinking. The universal laws rearranged things so that by the time I returned home, the timing was just right for the entry level requirements for that very university program. If I had entered previously at age eighteen, I would have been denied, but the timespan aged me just enough to be accepted since the grade requirement was lower for "mature" students. I had no idea until I applied; clearly, the universe waited to plant the seed of the idea in me, allowing the timing to unfold too.

You have a dream. Everyone has a purpose, and your intuition knows just what to do. Your job is to listen and take a step. Then one day, out of the blue, your intuition will reveal your truth, through the storms and all. In fact, in what feels like a storm forcing you to sit and wait with a little inner cleaning, is the Universe orchestrating the timing of your next awakening.

BE, DO, HAVE VS. HAVE, BE, DO

Zig Ziglar, author and speaker, is known for the above quote. He also said, "If you want happy, you must *be* happy and be the person who walks and talks happy to have happy." It isn't luck that brings success. It appears in the minds of those who have the opposite thinking. Dreams rarely come to fruition amid struggle. When Steve was unhappy, he received more unhappy, including his rock bottom shame of walking with a cane. The depression, the unhealthy choices, high sugars, cholesterol, blood pressure, and gout came on like a storm. His ocean needed cleaning, too, before he could see his dreams.

Steve dreamed of being a lead singer in a band. One afternoon, with a to-do list in hand, rehabilitated finger and all, he made a detour to grab lunch. Waiting for his food took some time, but he eventually made his way. What appeared to put him behind ended up being the perfect timing. As Steve hobbled through the aisles of the grocery store, he ran into his friend Robin. Catching up, Steve humbly explained his recent divorce and losing his way. He further detailed his desire to now fill his lonely hours by joining a band. Robin could not have been more amazed; he was searching for a lead singer for his band! This true story could not have been planned by humans; it was orchestrated by a Higher Power once Steve took a step. It is in taking a step that you step into the *be* to *do* and to *have* that allows all the pieces to fall into place.

When Steve joined the band, his authentic self emerged and healing took place. Motivated by his dream, today he not only follows a healthy lifestyle, but is also gout free and walks three miles a day. Steve is down forty pounds. He has written and recorded a song about his sons and calmed the fears that ignited the problems in the first place. Atonement heals once again!

LEARNING A NEW LANGUAGE TO MIND-FULL RESULTS

> "I believe that everything happens for a reason. People change so that you can learn to let go and sometimes good things fall apart so better things can fall together."
>
> — Marilyn Monroe

I rescued two small kittens assuming they would come in handy living on acreage with the potential of mice. Inherent in cats, of course, is the skill to catch mice, but for the better part of five years, they could not because my cats are blind. Still, their innate ability, despite barriers, didn't stop them from trying. Starting with toy mice and small adventures outside, they learned to strengthen their skills through their other senses. After a few years, my female cat seemed to catch on a little more. Sensing a mouse nearby, she would pounce, but without being able to see, the mouse could easily scurry away. Persistence eventually paid off, though, and she became a master mouser. Oddly enough, as soon as she caught on, it was as though the other one caught on. How? It wasn't by watching. Was there a connection on a conscious level? Did she teach him in some language?

Your soul is already in perfect health; it is innate in you, and your intuition is guiding you to align with it. If you are not experiencing optimal health, it is simply blocked by barriers you cannot see but that present themselves as disease. A blindness to your authentic self is much like the sun that never stops shining when it is blocked by clouds. Stay persistent, and play to your strengths; you are learning a new language you will master.

Just as the one cat learned, so did the other. When you teach, you learn, and when you learn, you teach. These tools are for everyone. They work even more so with children who already have flourishing imaginations. One study showed that children who apply their imagination with visionary tools consume less calories, eat healthier snacks, and have less tendency toward instant gratification and even less anxiety.

Remember when I was the "Plate Spinner"? It was at a time when my "R&R" was "Rules and Rigor," which led to hormonal upheaval.

I blamed my hormones. All I knew was the symptom level until becoming a life coach gently guided me to realizing I was creating the problem. Like a ball of stress, my body reciprocated.

After looking back to connect the dots, I am grateful the plates all fell in another chaotic storm. Spinning all those plates did not form the bond I have with my daughter today. I would not have learned a new language, known of my resilience, nor experienced the lessons of forgiveness on my prodigal return.

As Albert Einstein said, "You can't solve a problem with the same mind that created it." You can, however, solve a problem with a new mind. In hearing from a quietened, humble part of me in that storm, a light emerged from within. As Mary Morrissey says, "You cannot get to your dream, you must come from it." Ignite the same light within you.

CONNECTING THE DOTS

> "Each of us has an inner thermostat setting that determines how much love, success, and creativity we allow ourselves to enjoy. When we exceed our inner thermostat setting, we will often do something to sabotage ourselves, causing us to drop back into the old, familiar zone."
>
> — Gay Hendricks

Your relationships with food, money, people, and how you spend your time are all connected. Can you imagine fulfillment in all areas of your life? No more wondering when the other shoe will drop. Remember, those thoughts will be there, but with your awareness of thought patterns, you can connect the dots. As the quote above suggests, you have an inner thermostatic setting determining your level of fulfillment. Wondering when the shoe will drop is governing how long you allow yourself to marinade in joy. It will sabotage maintenance due to an underlying pattern of thinking from *temporary* success. All four areas (Health, Career, Relationships, Time/Money) can be disrupted. You might be looking forward to a romantic evening but hold thoughts like *Knowing us, we'll probably fight*, or *It's too expensive*, or *I'll eat too much*, and so on. An event most would envy, and movie scenes are based on, can be ruined by thought patterns before it even begins.

Fortunately, the flip side is also true. Once you notice your thoughts governing happiness, you can interrupt and repattern. If the one way is true, the other must be also. As Neville said in his book *The Power of Awareness*, "If you live right mentally, everything will be right. By a change of or in your mental diet, you can alter the course…unless there is a change in your mental diet, your personal history remains the same." Can you connect the dots looking back to when you changed your thinking and it brought you new results? If you succeed in one area, you can succeed in all areas. Listen to your intuitive guidance and continue to take steps, and connections will step toward you.

THE HEALER IN YOU

> "A healer does not heal you. A healer is someone who holds space for you while you awaken your own inner healer, so that you may heal yourself."
>
> — Maryam Hasnaa

Jennifer Jiménez, founder of the health and well-being division of the Brave Thinking Institute, suggests, "You have an inner physician. Your mind, body, and spirit speak to you. By tuning out your inner critic, you can tune into the inner healer in you."

Let *The Domino Diet Formula* serve you in creating the results you love in all areas of your life. You are a trendsetter opening new doors to possibilities and answers. Honing the formula will take you past the eighteen-mile mark, through invisible boundaries, to get even more from the unlimited supply in life. Be proud you invested the time to unleash the real you. It may have been a long path, but I trust it is a sustaining one. Your ocean needed to release debris and resentment amid blessings in the storms. Your results will continue to show you when it's time to reap or clean. When you experience emotional eating, heart disease symptoms, and so on, your body is speaking to you to get your attention, and to clean your thoughts. No more bailing water until you are burned out. You have tools to repair the leaks.

As long as you are breathing, there will be conflict, falling and rising, and a lot of rinse and repeat. The healing and recovery do quicken, though, with your sturdier structure. Like the bamboo tree, enjoy your eighteen feet of success held by the inner growth you invested in. Just by being here, you exemplify this. Your journey to optimal well-being isn't a race or a fad diet. It is lifelong, with a diet as a way of life. Health is for healing and healing is for health, starting with the mind.

When you feel unhealed energy, you have time before it becomes anything—feelings are only the midway point of the Domino Formula. Return to your thoughts—the first domino—and follow with your breath, the second domino, to switch on the third domino, which is your R&R hormonal cascade. The fourth domino will adjust your feelings and reciprocate your actions—the fifth domino. From there, your results will be influenced as the sixth domino falls with ease into the freedom of no longer dieting again. When you begin to live a life by design, you will want to extend your time with healthy eating, walking, and meditation. This is the right order and from the right place—all the dominoes do fall into place.

I admit it. I'm biased. While many suggest all four areas in your life (Health, Relationships, Career, Time/Money) are equal, I must confess I believe health is of the utmost importance. I believe you can have wealth, but without health, you cannot enjoy it. You can buy the Winnebago, but without health, you'll be selling it to pay your deductibles and co-pays. Relationships exist in times of disease, but with health, the richness is much more. I believe optimal health is the Holy Grail of a happier you, and using your intuition gives you access to the Fountain of Wisdom.

The other connection to be made in regards to the underlying theme of this book and Steve, Pamela, and others' successful results is how they embodied the message of health I discussed in the first chapter.

1. Nurture your body with the *right thoughts*—love your body and it will love you.
2. Nurture your body with the *right food*—fuel your body with whole, fresh, unprocessed foods.
3. Nurture your body with the *right people*—surround yourself with positive support.
4. Nurture your body with the *right environment*—fresh air, scenery, nature, aromas.

No longer in silos, they combined *Mind*-with healthy thoughts and invested in supports; *Body* with micronutrients healing on a cellular level while actively walking in nature or playing golf or meditating with yoga; and *Spirit* by following their intuition towards a dream.

I will end with the words of Joseph Murphy, author of the 1963 book *The Power of Your Subconscious Mind*. "Why is one man sad and another man happy? Why is one man joyous and prosperous and another man poor and miserable…. Why is one man healed of a so-called incurable disease and another isn't?" Is there an answer to these questions in the workings of your conscious and subconscious minds? There most certainly is. I do not know why some are dealt a hand of turmoil. I am aware of arguments against the notion of the mind as the root of all storms, but what I do know is the power of the mind has not been used or promoted to its full capacity.

Remember Leroy and Claire, who in 1967 were dealt a hand that changed the course of many lives? They stayed the course by leveraging their minds and rising above adversity. In *The Power of Your Subconscious Mind*, Joseph Murphy wrote, "Many are sound asleep because they do not know about this goldmine of infinite intelligence and boundless love within themselves. Whatever you want, you can draw forth." Murphy reminds us that a magnet can lift twelve times its own weight, but if demagnetized, "It will not even lift a feather." This invisible energy can draw to your magnified thoughts or become blocked by them. Leroy and Claire magnetized with their mind a true rags-to-riches story—riches of the richest kind. While many seek things outside themselves for wealth and health, they found the secret of the ages in the power of the mind.

Leroy and Claire will be celebrating their fifty-third wedding anniversary by the time this book is published. Together, they have three children and three grandchildren. The baby born in 1968 was me. I am forever grateful for their sacrifices and their evolving minds. They, along with the authors mentioned in this book and the *Nutritional Almanac*, influenced me and paved my path. And it was all from Dad's desire to provide for his family, and Mom, who traded in her youth for me. Like a rudder on a river, they have guided me to you.

What level of thinking will you and I embrace in a new era in the evolution of health using the mind, where there are no expenses or side effects? Heed the advice of the many sage authors quoted in this book. I'll leave you with this last one.

> "Keep your thoughts positive because your thoughts become your words. Keep your words positive because your words become your behavior. Keep your behaviors positive because your behaviors become your habits. Keep your habits positive because your habits become your values. Keep your values positive because your values become your destiny."
>
> — Mahatma Gandhi

DOMINO DIET FORMULA:

Thoughts⇒ Breath⇒ Hormones⇒ Feelings⇒ Actions⇒ **Results**⇒ … **Freedom!**

REFLECTIONS

1. What qualities would you most want in a mentor? List possible support you can benefit from and/or reach out to.

   _____

   _____

   _____

   _____

2. Describe a time when your still, small voice/intuition guided you and helped you hold to your goals despite all odds.

   _____

   _____

   _____

   _____

ACTION STEP

While taking three breaths in and calmly out as described previously, recall something you are grateful for and proud of. Now bring your dream to mind or read your vision from earlier action steps. Ask, "What step can I take from where I am now to move in the direction of my dream?" Take three minutes to jot down ideas, images, words, colors, and doodles. Looking at your ideas, determine which ones give you a sense of "electricity." Circle three to four and put on your calendar which days you can begin each step. Remember, inspiration and information alone do not produce transformation without your participation.

SUMMARY

You have arrived at the end after investing your time. You are now like a master builder with tools. Endeavor to move forward and keep taking one step at a time. The Universe will step toward you, and help you through the invisible boundaries. Then take another step—you never know what will emerge out of the blue and from within you. Below are a few *Domino Diet Formula* highlights.

* Refer to my website at www.TheDominoDiet.com for special access to resources and more....

DOMINO DIET HIGHLIGHTS

1. You have two minds; collaborate with both.
2. Positive thinking, affirmations, bring awareness to your thoughts.
3. Pause, breathe to the R&R to become your primary way of being.
4. Use sleep, calm, walking, music, and meditation to help balance hormones.
5. Balanced mind equals balanced hormones equals balanced eating.
6. Your awakening isn't a crisis; buy into your dream from your fountain of wisdom.
7. Positive words and stories equal a positive life.
8. Uncover hidden fear of success with paradigm shifts; transcend to a new era.
9. All macros belong—no more battles of separation.
10. Arm up with micros; fill up on what you need to nourish your body first.
11. Drive like a Ferrari, all four wheels balanced (health, career, love, time/money freedom).

12. Hook onto a dream to tow your desires; you are the driver and fear is behind you.
13. Vision, clarity, consistency.
14. Renew and release to find the authentic you.
15. Be, do, have vs. have, be, do.
16. Stay attuned, aligned, and intuitive.
17. Maintaining is a verb; it involves action.
18. Turn adversity into your university.
19. Diamonds are flawed but they still shine.
20. Your measures determine your rewards; let love guide you.

> "There is no diet that will do what eating healthy does."
>
> — Unknown

AFFIRMATION

I deserve a happy, rich, full, healthy life!

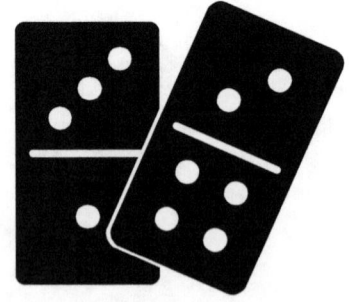

A FINAL NOTE

YOUR OPTIMAL WELL-BEING

> "Some people live ninety years; some people live one year ninety times."
>
> — Mary Morrissey

Now that you have read my book, I would like to personally congratulate you! A pat on the back is more than well deserved. You leaned in and played full out, allowing yourself to release, renew, and discover the true you. You have transformed and will continue to do so. It took courage to bust through the paradigms and make mindshifts. You are capable and worthy of anything you set your mind to. You've come this far and owe it to yourself to keep the momentum going. What can you do to sustain your efforts and continue onwards and upwards? What supports will help you stay fueled on your journey to a life you absolutely love?

Knowledge is power, and there is no limit to being, doing, and having in an empowering way. You can read all the books in the world, but if you do not apply the wisdom learned, you may lose the benefit. You are equipped now, and you have what it takes.

Using *The Domino Diet Formula*, I challenge you to list more steps you can implement in the next ninety days. If you need a reminder, refer to the list of "Ordinary to Extraordinary" tips in Chapter 18 to renew yourself. In fact, you are steps ahead since you have already started your journey toward a new you in 120 days. Keep going. New levels are being revealed to you from a healing mind. Become the best-energized version of yourself. On the ten lines below, list the steps you would love to take to discover your highest potential. After all, good is the enemy of great. Be great. Remember also to refer to my website, www.TheDominoDiet.com for tools such as The Domino Diet Workbook, The Domino Diet Journal/Food Journal, Calendar, affirmation cards, and more to help you to continue deepening your journey to self-love and freedom.

Ten Domino Diet Moments to Come

1. _____
2. _____
3. _____
4. _____
5. _____
6. _____
7. _____
8. _____
9. _____
10. _____

You have a formula that is with you wherever you go. You have learned the foundation of your results is your thoughts. Every idea imagined has the potential to become a reality. In fact, it already has in the world of energy. Become a match to the person who has those results already and they are yours. You get to choose your results by design rather than by default. As long as you are breathing, you are creating yourself one way or another. Align and attune to your conscious mind with your brilliant imagination in collaboration with your subconscious—the genie serving what you hold in your *vision* with consistency, clarity, and desire. It is yours.

When negativity rises up, *you* have access to a switch. Breathe with calm confidence to activate a cascade of hormone harmony. Be grateful for your hormones doing their job to serve you. Shed light on your fears and raise your love "hertz," feeling enlightened and turning your adversity into your university. Make progress instead of chasing perfection, and create a soft place to fall because a fall is inevitable for there to be a rise. Stay the course with the empowering question, "What would I love?" Your dreams, your optimal health, ideas, and steps are waiting to meet you as you step toward them, where love resides. Make a *you*-turn, release what no longer serves you, and replace it with what does. Let go of resentments by forgiving, healing from the inside out with love's emotions instead of anger's side effects, including emotional eating.

You have learned the real meaning of the word diet and why past diets did not last or provide healthy results. Healing is an inside job and not just at the symptom level. You have put the *"heal" back into "health"* with a healthy mind at the start. Now your diet is a way of life aligned to your body's needs, intuitively speaking. From your mind to micronutrients, armed and protected, you can skip your old diet thinking and be mindful of healing thinking with holistic, traditional, and alternative support.

If you apply the wisdom, knowledge, experience, skills, strategies, and techniques offered in this book, you will achieve what the title and subtitle promise. You will see more and more how everything is connected. Are you ready to reap the benefits in all areas of your life? The domino effect will fall into place in all areas, from health, wealth, love, and career to *freedom*!

I encourage you to contact me and share your successes! Send your questions and suggestions. There are more books ready to pour from me to you. I am there for you as a "Dietitian on a Mission," using my tools as a life coach, healer, and someone who has been there to support your journey. Tell me about you, your obstacles, your challenges, and your adversity so I can further help you. In fact, I would like to offer you a complimentary, no-obligation thirty-minute consultation to see how I and my team can best serve you.

My email address is info@TheDominoDiet.com, and my cell phone is (780)-814-2983, so please email me, or better yet, text me with your name and time zone, and we will schedule your complimentary consultation.

I wish you a "Wealth of Health"! I wish you a life you love with dreams to serve your optimal Abundant-Self! Your friend, The Authentic Inner Healer...

Karie Cassell

Author, Speaker, Life Mastery Coach, Dietitian, Healer

ABOUT THE AUTHOR

Karie Cassell is an internationally known professional author, keynote speaker, registered dietitian of more than thirty years, and certified life coach. Since the age of thirteen, she has been called to serve in wellness. After studying alternative medicine, she became a dietitian. Working in several areas in health and wellness, she specialized in heart disease, diabetes, and sports nutrition with the International Olympic Committee. She has served on the board and/or as chair for national and international health organizations. She discovered the real effect in holistically helping others find their optimal well-being, including a holistic approach. Karie's Life Coach Certification and specialty as a Life Mastery Consultant with the Brave Thinking Institute has provided a well-rounded approach to her current thriving private practice.

Along her journey, Karie discovered a passion for speaking in ways that reach masses of individuals, leaving them feeling renewed, inspired, and optimistic about their health and life endeavors. Her love of speaking took her to complete a Presentation Mastery certification with Toastmasters International, with distinctive awards for her level of achievement. As a result, Karie has become a sought-after speaker to thousands of audiences of all sizes and ages, on an international scale and on all platforms. Karie has helped over 100,000 people transform their health and well-being and has spoken to several thousands across 119 countries.

Karie has been featured on well-known media platforms such as FOX, CBS, NBC, and AP to a name a few. She has also been featured in magazines, newsletters, TV interviews, commercials, and success story spotlights.

She is an achiever in all "walks" of life, having completed full marathons and adventure races, traveled the world, been a successful business entrepreneur, and more importantly, a mom to her beautiful daughter Seanna and her bonus boys Tyler and Riley, and a wife to their dad Stephen.

> "It is lack of passionate direction to life that makes man fail of accomplishments.... We must move from thinking of the end to thinking from the end."
>
> — Neville

ABOUT KLC LIFEWISE COACHING

Karie Cassell offers private, invitation-only membership for you as a reader and anyone who wants to take charge of their life and become creators of their own dreams and destinies. From wealth to relationships, to your career and most definitely your health, if you want to make the connections and live a life filled with passion, review your options below:

1. Karie Cassell, Weekly Conference Call, and Webinars
2. VIP level Coaching and Supports
3. Classes, Workshops, Podcasts, and Blogs
4. Resources, Recipes, and Tools
5. E-books

Learn about special packages customized to your specific desires. Life Coaching, Wellness, Disease Management, Prevention, Sports Nutrition, and more are all available.

BOOK KARIE CASSELL TO SPEAK AT YOUR NEXT EVENT

When it comes to choosing a professional speaker for your next event, you will find no one more respected and uniquely qualified than Karie Cassell. Karie's experience as a Certified Life Coach with more than thirty years of studying wellness comes with a background as a Registered Dietitian. She brings an absolute passion as a "Dietitian on a Mission" to a professional speaking approach that will leave your audience or colleagues with a renewed passion for life. Her twist of humor and storytelling will teach you in ways you will not forget. You will leave saying "I never heard it that way before," and that's a promise!

Whether your audience is 10 or 10,000, in person or on webinar-type platforms, Karie delivers, nationally and internationally, customized inspirational messages. From her specialties in Health, Relationships, Wealth, and Career, she weaves her Life Coaching skills into her messages knowing your Well-Being spans all areas of your life.

Book Karie Cassell today!
www.TheDominoDiet.com
www.KLCLifeWise.com
info@theDominoDiet.com
Mobile: 780-814-2983

For Yoga and Wellness Coaching, Book Seanna Quinn today!

Mobile: 780-814-2983 / 587-202-5750
or yoga.quinn@gmail.com

"The natural healing force within each one of us
is the greatest force in getting well."

— Hippocrates

www.ingramcontent.com/pod-product-compliance
Lightning Source LLC
Chambersburg PA
CBHW051850170526
45168CB00001B/44